The Silicone Breast Implant Story: Communication and Uncertainty

The Silicone Breast Implant Story: Communication and Uncertainty

Marsha L. Vanderford
University of South FLorida

David H. Smith
Hong Kong Baptist University

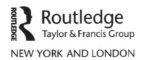
Routledge
Taylor & Francis Group

NEW YORK AND LONDON

First Published by
Lawrence Erlbaum Associates, Inc., Publishers
10 Industrial Avenue
Mahwah, New Jersey 07430

Transferred to Digital Printing 2009 by Routledge
270 Madison Avenue New York, NY 10016
2 Park Square Milton Park, Abingdon Oxon OX14 4RN

Cover design by Gail Silverman

Library of Congress Cataloging-in-Publication Data

The silicone breast implant story : communication and
uncertainty / Marsha L. Vanderford, David H. Smith.
p.   cm.
Includes bibliographical references and index.
ISBN 0-8058-1706-9 (c : alk. paper). — ISBN 0-8058-
1707-7 (p : alk. paper)
1. Breast implants—Complications. 2. Sili-
cones—Toxicology. 3. Health risk communication. 4.
Breast implants—Complications—Public opinion. I.
Smith, David H. II. Title.
[DNLM: 1. Mammaplasty. 2. Implants, Artificial. 3.
Women—psychology. 4. Communication 5. Silicones.
WP 910 V232s 1996]
RD539.8.V36 1996
628.1'9059—dc20
DNLM/DLC
for Library of Congress   96-13566
                                                          CIP

Publisher's Note
The publisher has gone to great lengths to ensure the quality
of this reprint but points out that some imperfections in the
original may be apparent.

CONTENTS

Preface

Our title is meant to illustrate that the idea of the story plays a special role in this book. We found the narrative concept helpful both in doing our research and in interpreting its results. We suggest that our readers also adopt that perspective as they read our work. They will find that a series of stories follow. The topics differ and the ways of telling them change, especially as the research methods vary, but together the smaller narratives combine into one larger story of an important controversy in health. We hope readers will see the importance of the separate stories in the various chapters and that they will also perceive the overall narrative of how communication shapes the individual perceptions of health and government and social policy concerning health care.

Chapter 1 tells our story as authors and sketches the overall narrative of breast implants and silicone gel. Chapters 2 and 3 present the accounts of women who believe their silicone gel implants have made them ill. Chapter 4 tells the stories of women who are pleased with their implants. Chapter 5 presents the accounts of doctors from various specialties who differed, even publicly, about the safety and efficacy of silicone gel breast implants. Chapters 6 and 7 analyze the stories in the media. Chapter 6 focuses on narratives about the safety and risk of implants. Chapter 7 looks at the stories that vilified plastic surgeons. Chapter 8 tells the story of Dow Corning's failed public relations efforts to counter negative media accounts. Chapter 9 uses survey results to capture how women in general were constructing their own stories of the implant controversy. Chapter 10 interprets the previous narratives and offers an explanation of what happened in the controversy.

We began work on the silicone breast implant controversy because it generated ethical questions for our plastic surgery colleagues. From that beginning, our inquiry broadened to the communication questions involved. At the core of the controversy was the need of people to act amid uncertainty about the health risks involved. That need, to weigh action in the midst of uncertain risk, characterizes a large number of health issues. The attempts of patients, physicians, drug manufacturers, and others to seek and provide both information and influence made communication central to those issues. Consequently, the questions explored here will interest a diverse group of readers.

Because breast implants are inherently linked to images of femininity, beauty, and self-esteem, we hope our book is helpful to those interested in women's health issues. The indepth personal interviews we conducted with women who had implants reveal how women manage their health and self-concepts. Additionally, the differences revealed in how they interacted with their physicians adds to a growing body of literature concerning women's experiences in the health care system.

We also see our work as relevant to the interests of plastic surgeons, in particular, and to physicians, in general. As the medical profession struggles with its identity amid changes in public attitudes, government regulation, and medical practice, our findings concerning media portrayals of doctors and medical devices may be telling. In addition, physicians may find breast implants a helpful case study for considering the different ways that their colleagues make health decisions across specialties.

Clearly we hope this volume is helpful to those interested in how we communicate about our health in public and private forums. We are scholars in health communication. This study has revealed how interrelated public information and private decisions are and how closely media and interpersonal relationships fit. Tracing one medical issue across interpersonal, organizational, public relations, and mediated forums has given us the opportunity to see the multiple ways those communication channels overlap and inform one another.

We have not attempted to weigh and judge the medical evidence about the safety and efficacy of silicone gel breast implants. That effort is beyond our expertise. But we have learned much about those who, because they had chosen to have implant surgery, were faced with uncertainty about their health. Some resolved their uncertainty by blaming their implants and their doctors for illness experiences. Others dismissed the publicity about implant danger as unproved. Still others were influenced by the publicity to worry about a decision that had previously caused them no concern. Those interested in the human dimension of what it was like to be an implant patient or a doctor caring for such patients will find much of interest in what follows.

Throughout our work we were dependent on the generosity of a number of other people, many of whom we promised anonymity in return for their cooperation. We cannot, therefore, name those patients, physicians, and others who assisted us by talking freely about their experiences and making it possible for us to obtain access to people and materials. They have our sincere gratitude and we hope they will see themselves as, in a way, authors of the material that follows. They need not accept responsibility for our conclusions, but without their help we would have been unable to put together this whole project.

There are others whose help we can acknowledge. Chuck Grant, Keith Cherry, Karen Cunningham, Rebecca Hemmick, Belicia Efros, Yvonne Bissonnette, and Elaine Kwok gave significant assistance with the scholarly details. Andrea Davis, Liz Melton, Olga Torres, Monica Chau, Mimi Yip, Trinh Thompson, and Mavis Green provided invaluable secretarial support. We would especially like to thank

Barbara Orchard. She was truly a partner in completing the final manuscript through multiple editions, far more than she had counted on.

The Department of Internal Medicine in the persons of its founding chair, Roy Behnke, and the director of its division of Medical Ethics and Humanities, Robert Walker, provided support and time to write. The Communication Department and its former chair, Terrance Albrecht, also gave key support and allowed us time to write. Willard Harris was of special assistance. We could not have completed the project without the friendship, cooperation, and encouragement of our colleagues in the Divisions of Plastic Surgery and Rheumatology. They were interested in our work, but let us do it our way and draw our own conclusions. To our friends and colleagues at both South Florida and Hong Kong Baptist, we owe great thanks for their special tolerance of our obsession with this topic. They never told us to shut up though they must have felt like it.

Hollis Heimbouch encouraged us to do the book and to try to write it in a more readable way than is sometimes true of scholarly prose. Teri Thompson was always positive and encouraging. Her suggestions helped make the book better. Tonja Olive gave valuable assistance to us throughout our work and was a real partner in several of the studies we undertook. As a student interested in women's affairs, particularly women's health, she quite properly saw this issue as as important women's health issue attracting considerable attention.

We each would like to acknowledge the loving support, interest, and friendship of a few without whose faith and counsel we could not have completed this work. David A. Carter, Ellen Stevens, Kathleen Heide, Eldra Solomon, Fran Knowles, Lisa Day, Beverley Shovar, Carolyn Gross, and James Eison were vital to Marsha. Dave thanks especially Harry Irwin, David Pendleton, and Paul Arnston. Jeanne Smith read every chapter, made useful suggestions, listened with infinite and loving patience, provided unconditional support, and photographed the Tampa attorney's billboard soliciting clients with implants, which appears later. She was, as always, a gift.

A work like this requires special trust and willingness to accept help between its authors. Distance places special demands on that relationship. We thank each other for being tolerant and accepting. We also thank the inventor of the telephone, fax, and E-mail for making our long distance cooperation possible. Those devices have not yet reached perfection, but we would have been lost without them.

Marsha L. Vanderford
David H. Smith

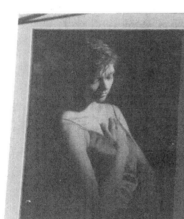

1

THE AUTHORS' STORY:
A PROJECT WITH A LIFE OF ITS OWN

It all started in 1991, with a telephone call from a friend in the plastic surgery division of our medical school. He was worried about an ethical problem and wanted to discuss it with someone who taught medical ethics. We knew him to be a good doctor. One of the authors, Dave, had worked with him on a program about ethics and the treatment of patients in the burn unit, and on a subcommittee to design a human values program for the medical school. He was the kind of colleague we liked and wanted to help.

The problem, as he explained over the telephone, was that, even though they thought there was no medical benefit in doing so, he and a colleague had decided to remove silicone gel breast implants from several women who had requested removal. These plastic surgeons believed that there was no danger to women's health from silicone gel breast implants. Nonetheless, they felt that the requests for removal were reasonable extensions of patients' rights to control their own bodies.

As we talked to our plastic surgeon colleagues, we discovered that a number of plastic surgeons were unwilling to remove implants. Those doctors argued that in the absence of good scientific evidence pointing to danger from silicone gel breast implants, the inherent surgical risks could not be justified. Hence, the surgery for removal would be unethical, exposing patients to risks without potential benefits. Our plastic surgeon colleagues had reached a different conclusion based on their commitment to patient autonomy. Our colleagues were criticized by other members of the plastic surgery community. As a result of the conflict, our colleagues wanted to think through the issue with someone familiar with medical ethical issues. We ultimately reassured them that we thought their removals were ethically defensible under the autonomy principle. If a woman could consent to have implants inserted, accepting that surgical risk because of her own belief in their benefit, surely she could consent to their removal because she now believed in the benefit of having them out. We felt it would be untenable to require a woman to retain a foreign object in her body that she felt was harming her because no surgeon agreed to remove it. Removal, although still believed to be unwise by many plastic surgeons, is no longer ethically controversial. Many surgeons will perform the procedure.

However, that was not the end of the problem, only its beginning. As we listened to our colleagues' description of difficulties the women requesting removal had faced, we learned that another of our faculty colleagues, a rheumatologist, had come to believe that there was a connection between silicone gel implants and certain disease symptoms. The syndrome was first called autoimmune disease, then human adjuvant disease, and finally connective tissue disease. This rheumatologist had seen enough individual cases, where women with implants had rheumatological symptoms, that he concluded there might be a connection. He advised some patients to consider the possibility of removing their implants. When those patients' own plastic surgeons refused to remove the implants, the rheumatologist referred them to his faculty colleagues in the Division of Plastic and Reconstructive Surgery. These were the patients whose implants had been removed, and who continued to make requests for such removal.

Our conversation with the plastic surgeons gave us our first glimpse of what was to become a major focus of our study and research. We heard, for the first time, about women who cared enough about their appearance to pay the costs of silicone gel breast implants, yet later decided on removal, despite the clear advice that their appearance would be far worse than before the implants. We got the first glimmer of differences of opinion among physicians across specialty lines and even within the plastic surgery community itself. We heard the first hints of the painful personal stories of women who thought their implants had made them ill.

Because we are primarily interested in communication and the sense people create out of experiences and messages, we wondered how these patients would make meaning out of what had happened to them. We also were committed to the idea that the details necessary to properly understand ethical problems in medicine come from the stories of those people involved. We had listened to the stories of the plastic surgeons about the ethical conflict and the criticism from their colleagues. We thought it would be wise to hear from several of the patients.

With the help of our plastic surgery colleagues, and with patient consent, we interviewed four women. We asked them to tell us their stories. As scholars, we believe narrative to be an important perspective from which to understand human experience. As a result, we used unstructured interview techniques to assist the women in unfolding the stories of their own experiences. What we first heard from our initial four interviews later became familiar. Having sought to improve their appearance with implants and initially being pleased with the results, the patients later experienced symptoms they finally attributed to the implants. These symptoms were debilitating, but the doctors they visited failed to recognize any syndrome or disease. The doctors then sought other causes, often psychological causes in the women themselves. The patients became frustrated with physicians and the medical system in general. They felt they had to become their own health advisors. They looked to media information and other women as guides.

From the very first, we were struck by the pain and difficulty these patients had endured in their quest to understand what was happening inside their bodies, by their frustration in dealing with doctors unable to find ways to help them, and by their desperate search for hope and meaning. We determined that this was a project worth examining in more detail and set out on what became a series of studies about communication surrounding the breast implant controversy.

AN INTRODUCTION TO THE STUDIES

When we began, we anticipated one study collecting the stories of women who believed their implants had made them ill. We thought hearing how these women interpreted their experiences would tell us something interesting about health communication. Our rheumatology colleagues and our plastic surgery colleagues were very helpful and facilitated our contact with women who had breast implants and health problems. The doctors asked their patients if they would be willing for us to request interviews. We were able to approach those who said "yes," obtain their consent, and record interviews, which sometimes ran more than 2 hours.

We became increasingly aware of the disagreement among physicians of different specialties about whether silicone gel breast implants were related to connective tissue disease. We decided that it would be necessary to talk with doctors from a number of specialties to learn how they came to these conclusions and why they assessed the information available in such different ways. We were also interested in doctors' responses to the patients because we had begun to hear patients describe what they felt were unsatisfactory conversations with their physicians. Doctors were being blamed for poor communication as well as lack of scientific knowledge. So we arranged to talk with both rheumatologists and plastic surgeons to try to understand their differing perceptions.

During this time, we learned that a group of plastic surgeons had filed a formal complaint with the Department of Professional Regulation in the state of Florida asking that disciplinary action be taken against one of the rheumatologists on our faculty for telling women that their symptoms were related to silicone gel implants. In the view of the complaining plastic surgeons, there was no evidence supporting the rheumatologist's conclusion. They argued that this was poor medical practice and should be restricted by those regulating the licensing of physicians in the state of Florida. The complainants also included criticism of the University plastic surgeons for the removal of implants. We thus decided that we needed to interview community physicians as well as University physicians. Despite the strong disagreement between community plastic surgeons and physicians at the University, and despite our clear identification with the University and its medical school, community physicians were generous with their time and willing to talk to us about their perspectives.

As weeks and months in 1991 passed, the volume of attention to the breast implant issue in the press increased dramatically. We became increasingly curious as to how this issue was being described by the press in contrast to the way it was being described by the physicians and patients with whom we talked. We began to clip articles from the local papers. As these accumulated, we decided that we needed a systematic review of the press coverage and began to collect all the relevant articles from the *St. Petersburg Times*, the daily newspaper in our metropolitan area having the largest circulation. The *Times* is considered to be a good newspaper and works hand in hand with its majority owner, the Poynter Institute for Media Studies, which strives to study and disseminate high journalistic standards. We searched the *Readers' Guide to Periodical Literature* back 30 years to locate all the articles on the subject in popular magazines that would have been available to women readers in the Tampa Bay area. We went to a newsstand each week and looked through all the women's magazines and supermarket tabloids for any article related to breasts or breast implants. When we found one, we added it to our collection. We added occasional articles from the *Tampa Tribune*, the other major metropolitan daily newspaper in our area. Although we are not sure we got all of those, we believe we clipped most of them during the time period we studied. Friends gave us articles from out of town newspapers including the *Wall Street Journal*, the *New York Times*, and the *Los Angeles Times*. In this way, we assembled a collection of press coverage that could reasonably be expected to represent what a woman living in the Tampa Bay area might have had the opportunity to read about the silicone breast implant issue.

We knew that the television coverage of the controversy was also important. A number of the women with problems told us about the key role television had played in their self-diagnosis and commitment to take action about their implants. *Face to Face with Connie Chung* (Lack, 1990) was mentioned time and time again. Our interviewees said that it was hearing other women talk about their symptoms that made them decide the implants were causing their illnesses. Even doctors saw the television coverage as important. They told us about the large number of calls they got from former patients after shows like *Connie Chung* wondering if they should be worried about their implants. Two obstetrician/gynecologists said that they had obtained most of their information about the implant controversy from the news coverage, particularly television, rather than from scientific journals.

We then decided we needed to collect television coverage, but it was much more difficult to obtain than news clippings. We had to be watching the right channel at the right moment to catch local stories and get the video recorder going with a fresh tape. We were seldom able to do this. Friends and colleagues were able to provide us with some examples, but ultimately, we decided to order copies of the major network news broadcast coverage of the silicone gel breast implant issue from the archives at Vanderbilt University. Our sample of television coverage was primarily national network news and did not contain a representative sample of local programs. However, the national telecasts were broadcast on our local channels and were available to those viewing the news in the Tampa Bay area.

The media coverage of the problems some women attributed to their implants was dramatic and compelling. Many of our friends, relying on those dramatic stories, told us how dangerous they thought implants must be. But little was said about the women with implants who were healthy and satisfied with their implants. They seemed to be less prominent in the news. One local station, perhaps in an attempt to balance its coverage, followed an intense statement by a woman who believed her implants were killing her, with a brief interview with a bikini-clad woman on the beach. The woman stated that she really liked her implants. However, her frivolous demeanor and provocative dress created an image that hardly seemed fair to serious women with implants, maybe not even fair to the woman whose 10 seconds of fame were obviously edited from a longer conversation. We wondered how other women with implants were reacting to the explosion in publicity about problems with devices they, too, carried in their bodies. Were they made anxious by the reports of those who said they were ill? To answer these questions, we decided to interview women with implants who were not experiencing symptoms to see if they viewed implants differently from those who felt themselves to be ill. This actually proved more difficult than finding patients who felt their implants were giving them problems. After all, women without problems were not likely to present themselves to doctors to talk about the issue.

Obtaining the opportunity to interview these patients presented a difficult problem in confidentiality. We did not feel we could ask physicians to give us the names of women who had implants because these patients might not want anyone to know that they had undergone the procedure. Most of us want some privacy concerning our medical care and, given the personal nature of breast implant surgery, it was likely that these women would want even more confidentiality than most. We were able to find several plastic surgeons who were willing to have staff members call women with implants to determine if they would be willing for us to contact them. We were then given those names, but only after the women had consented to be interviewed. We were able to interview several women in this way. We were also able to obtain the names of women from former interviewees who knew friends who had implants and were willing to ask those friends if we could contact them.

However, the press coverage was available to all women, not just those with implants. If it had influenced women with implants so dramatically, was it also influencing women without implants? Would women who did not have implants, but who had read the papers or watched TV news stories react like the women we had interviewed? How were women without implants interpreting all the dramatic publicity and controversy? What might they be learning from their friends who had implants with either positive or negative experiences? How were they placing this information in the context of health care generally and specifically in the context of women's health? We decided in order to obtain that kind of information, we needed to survey a representative sample of women about their information and attitudes toward silicone gel breast implants. Drawing on the interviews we had conducted and on the news articles, we developed and tested a questionnaire.

The process of completing the survey proved instructive. Because we were doing this study without funding, we could not simply hire a research firm to undertake the survey for us, nor could we buy a mailing list, employ interviewers, and supervise the interview process. We discovered that the day of the shopping mall intercept study is over, because private corporations now contract with every large shopping mall for the right to do surveys within their complexes. Based on the large numbers of people who go to the biggest flea market in our area, we decided this would provide a real opportunity to conduct a survey. We further decided that offering a free lottery ticket as a reward for completing the questionnaire would be a low-cost way to provide an incentive for women to do so. We reasoned that lottery tickets would cost us only a dollar each, but offered the illusion of a much larger payoff and would, therefore, provide a strong incentive. We rented a space at the Wagon Wheel Flea Market, made signs, printed questionnaires, bought lottery tickets, and arrived early and eager. We failed, however, to do what good social scientists should have done. We had not studied the behavior of people at flea markets before we set up our booth and began to attempt to collect data.

What we discovered, as thousands of people walked by us without stopping to complete the questionnaire, was that people at flea markets develop a strategy for dealing with the hundreds of booths they might visit. They can only take time to look over what is in a few. Shoppers, thus, engage in a kind of a scanning and selection procedure. They do not break stride as they walk by. Instead, they look ahead, scanning the next few booths they will pass for clues that a booth might be of interest. Because many of the booths feature hawkers trying to lure potential customers inside, we often failed to capture the visitors' eye contact. They did not care about free lottery tickets. We spent 8 hours at a flea market, which probably had 20,000 visitors that Saturday, and obtained two completed questionnaires! We ended up with a large number of unused lottery tickets and a lesson in the importance of studying the context in which you plan to do your research before you undertake it.

With our flea market experience gone but not forgotten, we then decided that the only way to collect this information was through the cooperation of intact groups. We, therefore, contacted a number of women's groups, including the Legal Secretaries Association, Women in Construction, and Business and Professional Women. With their cooperation, we were able to obtain 400 completed questionnaires. The sample is not representative of all women in our area; the respondent's education and income levels are significantly above the average. The results may nonetheless represent those women who are able to afford the cost of silicone gel breast implants. The data from this survey enabled us to check attitudes of women likely to have been exposed to the media coverage we were examining. We were also able to ask these women about their use of media, at the same time, we learned what they knew and thought about the silicone gel breast implant controversy.

Meanwhile, Tonja Olive began to look at the response of the Dow Corning Wright Company, the most prominent manufacturer of implants, to criticism from the press, plaintiffs in the courts, and the Food and Drug Administration (FDA).

As a graduate student at the University of South Florida, Tonja had become interested in the intersections of public relations, women's studies, health communication, and rhetoric. She obtained public relations materials from Dow Corning, looked at the press coverage of its actions, and completed an analysis of the company's crisis communication. Her study became the basis of chapter 8, "Vilification Stories: The Fall of Dow Corning."

The project seemed to have a life of its own. As we became involved in one aspect, we discovered others that needed to be considered, and so additional studies were undertaken. We initially had only been interested in the stories of women who felt they were ill, but we soon found ourselves trying to complete a series of studies that gave us a variety of perspectives, using diverse methods. We looked at the press coverage, for example, first, simply in terms of the orientation of the content. Was it pro-implant, anti-implant, or balanced in its coverage? Although that effort was interesting, we felt we missed much of the richness in the coverage. We then went back to analyze the articles for their narrative qualities. We used a similar way of looking at the interviews, trying to tease out the stories being told by the interviewees as a way of understanding how they had constructed meaning out of their experiences. In the interviews, we constantly pushed subjects to give us examples and anecdotes that would illustrate what they were thinking. These became the grist for our analytic mill.

When you are immersed in a subject like this, all kinds of experiences become related to it. Women's breasts, of course, are heavily associated with gender differences and sexuality in our society. Dave, when asked what he was working on, often received jibes and joking remarks in response, as if a man could not have only a scholarly interest in the topic. If he tried to help the jokers see the serious importance of the issue in health communication about risk, some people became uncomfortable. It appears that once a topic has been defined as a source of fun, some people have difficulty seeing the subject as a serious issue. On the other hand, a number of women, hearing of the research, wanted to talk about their concerns and experiences. At one point in the study, a secretary noticed Dave was photocopying materials on implants and volunteered highly personal information. They had been acquaintances for a number of years, but had never talked much about their personal lives. When she learned of his research interest, the secretary told Dave about her decision to have implants, her husband's reaction, and her own feelings about them.

Reasoning that women would usually feel more comfortable talking about sexually related topics with another woman, Marsha did most of the interviews with women. She developed a strong identification with them. It was difficult to hear their stories without empathizing with the pain they had experienced. On one occasion, she was interviewing a group of five women who had come from Denver to Tampa to visit a rheumatologist when one, quite unexpectedly, pulled up her sweatshirt to show the results of her implant removal. Where breasts and nipples had been, there were only ugly scars and a concave chest. At the sight of the mutilation, Marsha reflexively threw her arms across her own chest in a kind of unconscious defense of her breasts and her personhood.

It was not a project from which we could remain detached. It mattered too much to too many people. We found it easy to identify with nearly everyone we talked to, regardless of their opinions and experiences. The women we interviewed seemed to be reasonable people. We believed them when they said they had suffered. We also believed those who had no trouble. We believed each group of doctors even when they disagreed with one another. Some of these people were angry and found some of the others unreasonable. Yet, each seemed sincere to us, convinced that their interpretations of experience were valid. All were seriously concerned and willing to help us. We believed in their sincerity and were able to express the arguments of each group. This sometimes made us uncomfortable. Those we talked to seemed to regard us as medical experts. They wanted to know whether we thought implants were safe. This query came from women being interviewed, from reporters from whom we sought information, and from friends and colleagues. When we spoke about our survey findings to one of the women's groups that had completed questionnaires for us, the first question was whether we thought implants were safe. Of course, we are not medical experts. Even if we had opinions, those opinions ought not to carry weight in a scientific discussion of health risks.

Sometimes, we felt obliged to explain a contrary view to individuals who passionately agreed with a particular side of the controversy. Invariably, that was interpreted as meaning we agreed with their adversaries. Following one public presentation, Dave attempted to explain an opposing view to an excellent news columnist who believed silicone was causing illness. After Dave's comments, the columnist responded, "I can see you agree with the plastic surgeons." Conversely, when we presented a report on news coverage about silicone implants to a group of plastic surgeons, some audience members reacted angrily. In the question-answer period following the presentation, we found ourselves defensive on behalf of the media. We did not necessarily support either perspective. We saw multiple points of view. Neither of us decided to have implants, but we became more understanding of the reasons women had for getting them. No one wanted us to be detached and objective.

We were involved in other ways. People told us jokes about silicone gel breast implants. Some were even funny. One day while driving along the freeway, we looked up to see billboards, placed around the community by a trial attorney, featuring an attractive woman wearing a satin chemise and a worried look. "Silicone scared?" the billboards asked, and suggested calling this attorney for help.

As people began to learn of our work, we began to get long phone calls from some of the *Silicone Sisters*. Silicone Sisters was the name given by the local press to support groups for concerned women. They wanted to tell us their stories, to make sure we understood. Tonja attended several of the support group meetings. One news reporter who had been covering the topic talked to us at great length about her perceptions.

One morning the newspaper greeted us with an ad from Dow Corning announcing a hotline to call for information. We called, only to be answered by a machine asking us to leave a name and address. A number of weeks later we received information from them. A news article alerted us to another hot line, this one offering advice and referrals to lawyers for women who were worried. It was established by a nurse–legal aid in our community who, we were told, received hundreds of calls. As we talked with women who had undergone subcutaneous mastectomies in the hope of preventing breast cancer, we became more intensely aware of the nature of that epidemic and the fear that breast cancer inspires in women. In short, this project was not one we could easily put aside. Even when we turned to other pursuits, it jumped out everywhere we looked.

What drove us throughout, in addition to our curiosity, was a concern for two aspects of this particular issue. First, it is a women's health issue. The women's movement in particular, and large numbers of women in general, have been critical of the way doctors have treated them. When we talk informally to women about their health care, we often hear them say that they do not think their physicians listen to them or take them seriously. They say that male doctors often act as if their problems are only emotional, or even hysterical. These women resent the medical system for not treating women fairly. The women who expressed resentment did not all consider themselves to be feminists. Women who, in most other ways are conservative, happy with the society and their role in it, share anger about not being taken seriously by doctors. Revelations about the absence of female subjects in major medical studies lend credence to the neglect of women in the health care system. The fact that the Center for Disease Control (CDC) has established a positive program for the collection of data on women's health is evidence of the validity of that claim. Of course, the women's movement concerns more than health issues. But for many women, physicians are prototypical stereotypes of the male authority, which they feel has oppressed them. Few plastic surgeons are women.

The silicone gel breast implant controversy seemed to us to have much in common with a number of other women's health issues, such as the use of estrogen to prevent osteoporosis and the treatment of premenstrual syndrome (PMS). By trying to understand this controversy in more depth, we might develop a better understanding of how doctors and patients communicate about women's health issues in general, and how the press and the public respond.

In addition, this is an issue involving uncertainty, ambiguity, and risk. In selecting medical treatment, after discussions with physicians, most patients weigh risk-benefit information. However, we are not sure that risk information is always discussed directly and openly in doctor–patient conversations. Most doctors inform patients about the chances of some side effects versus the probability of treatment success. Medications have side effects and, sometimes, heavy interactions with one another. How do people assess and weigh those probabilities? People are usually informed before they consent to procedures, but what do the risk data say to them?

Public health campaigns and the press give probability information in an attempt to help us deal with medical uncertainties. Yet, the reporting of that information often leaves us confused. We are perplexed by relative risk data. What does it mean that men who took vitamin A had a lower death rate? Sometimes it seems that everything causes cancer. Information seems contradictory, and at best, ambiguous and uncertain. We are interested in how people create meaning about their health and about actions that might benefit them when faced with that ambiguity and uncertainty. Do they attend to data or are other influences more prominent?

This intellectual concern about risk, as well as a concern about women's health, supplemented our natural curiosity and the excitement about being involved in what had become a public controversy. In the process, we believe we learned a great deal that is useful to us and we hope will be useful to our readers as this book unfolds. To put our work in context, we begin with some of what we learned about the history of breast implants. Then we turn to the various studies we performed, how we did them, and what we think we learned from them.

A BRIEF HISTORY

Although this project is not a history of breast implants, some historical context is helpful in understanding the contemporary controversy. For centuries, clothing has been designed to enhance the prominence of breasts. The addition of the medical profession to the effort apparently began early in the 20th century. Guthrie (1994) mentioned medical reports of lumps and hardness from wax injections as early as 1912, and said occasional reports of complications from wax injection continued to appear into the 1960s.

The plastic, silicone, was first developed in the 1930s. It is a polymer that can be manufactured as a liquid, a gel, or a solid (Bruning, 1992). Following World War II, doctors began injecting small amounts of silicone into the body as an aid to filling depressions and offsetting wrinkles. In Japan, prostitutes wanting to appeal to occupying American GIs began to have silicone injected into their breasts. However, bad side effects occurred. The silicone did not stay where it was injected, lumps that felt like tumors developed, breasts hardened, and more serious health problems developed for a number of these women (Vasey & Feldstein, 1993). The silicone used was not generally sterile and was often adulterated with paraffin, wax, olive oil, or motor oil. The media reported that the silicone was sometimes mixed with industrial strength transformer coolant (Goodman, 1992). The FDA banned silicone injections in the United States, but a number of American women had them nonetheless. They, too, experienced problems.

Surgeons then tried using women's own fatty tissue to enlarge their breasts, but that proved unsatisfactory. The tissue lumped or was absorbed into the body. Ocean sponges became the next possibility. Medical researchers hoped the sponges would compress somewhat like natural breast tissue, but the body's immune response rejected them. Artificial sponges were tried, but they developed scar tissue and hardened. Something like a ball of bubble wrap was tried in hopes that the movement of the air in the bubbles would have a natural feel. However, like bubble wrap, the individual cells would occasionally break with a loud popping sound when squeezed. Changes in airplane cabin pressure also caused popping. Additionally, infection rates were high (Guthrie, 1994).

Dow Corning introduced a new device in 1965. It sealed silicone gel in a sack of silicone sheeting so that it could not escape, lose its shape, or migrate through the body. The implants could be made and kept sterile. (See chap. 8 for additional detail about Dow Corning's implant development and about the evolution of implants.)

Because silicone is believed to be inert, it is used widely in medical devices, shunts, drains, catheters, artificial valves and joints, pacemaker coatings, and penile and testicular implants. It is the lubricant used in syringes. To the plastic surgeons who had seen so many unsuccessful attempts to find a safe and effective means of breast augmentation and replacement, silicone gel breast implants were a breakthrough. Silicone gel implants rapidly became the industry standard and remained so until the FDA limited their use in 1992.

Over the years following Dow Corning's first implants, manufacturers continued to try to improve the shape of the implants and the consistency of the gel. A sack within a sack design called the *double lumen* came on the market. Because the body sometimes treats the implant as a foreign object surrounding it with scar tissue, a capsular contracture can form, making the breast hard. Authorities disagree on how often this happens, but the manufacturers tried various modifications to limit its occurrence, including changes in the implant's external texture. A coating of polyurethane was added to some implants. Throughout these changes, the silicone gel implant remained the most popular type of breast implant, and its use steadily climbed.

In the 1970s, saline-filled implants began to appear. Early problems with leakage and consequent deflation slowed its adoption, but gradually more plastic surgeons began to consider it an alternative. The inflatable implant became the saline implant of choice. A partially filled implant is placed in the body and then filled to the desired size and fullness by injecting additional saline into a valve, which then seals. The bag into which the saline is placed is made of silicone. Saline implants improved over time, but many plastic surgeons still believe that silicone gel implants provide a more natural look and feel in artificially enhanced breasts.

Implants were not regulated as medical devices by the U.S. government until 1976, when Congress included them with other medical devices to be regulated by the FDA. Because they were already on the market they were allowed to remain without the evidence of safety being submitted by their manufacturers, as would have been necessary for a new product. Implants were not singled out for such "grandfathering." A number of other devices were treated similarly because no evidence was available showing harm.

In 1982, the FDA decided to change the classification of implants and to require evidence of safety, but this process did not take place quickly. Not until 1988 did the agency finally tell the manufacturers to submit safety data, and it gave them 2 ½ years to do so.

Meanwhile, the beginnings of what was to become a major public controversy had emerged. The outer shell of the implant was supposed to be impervious to migration of the gel, but evidence gradually accumulated showing that the gel could "bleed" through the outer shell and go into the body. Some women had experienced problems with their implants; ruptures, leaking, and hardening were most frequent. Allegations were raised that the gel that bled or leaked caused illness in some women. The range of symptoms attributed to silicone leakage was broad. A number of rheumatological conditions were prominently mentioned: rheumatoid arthritis, scleroderma, and lupus among them. Complaints about these problems reached the FDA.

In 1990, Congressman Ted Weiss held hearings before the House Committee on Human Resources. A number of women testified about their problems, among them Sybil Goldrich, who later formed a support and advocacy group called Command Trust (Bruning, 1992). Weiss brought pressure to bear on the FDA to speed up the silicone implant review process. *Face to Face with Connie Chung* (Lack, 1990) was devoted to the issue in November 1990. That program, and its rebroadcast a year, later generated an avalanche of response from women now worried about their implants.

In 1991, the FDA held hearings on charges that polyurethane covered implants, the Même and the Replicon, could be dangerous because polyurethane could break down into a chemical, 2 TDA, which caused liver cancer in some laboratory animals. The FDA scientific advisory panel called for the manufacturers to conduct research on the possibility of this happening in humans. However, the hope that these implants would eliminate hardening had not been achieved, and the manufacturers withdrew them from the market rather than carry out the research. Much of the presumed association of implants with cancer might be traceable to the polyurethane implant story.

In November 1991, the FDA called on its scientific panel to evaluate the evidence of safety submitted by the manufacturers. The panel concluded that, although no evidence of danger existed, more evidence was needed to establish safety. The panel called for further research.

The same month Mariann Hopkins was awarded a very large settlement by a California jury. She claimed she suffered immune system difficulties because of her implants that had ruptured. However, her doctor testified that Hopkins had the symptoms before she had implants. In the process of discovery, documents were obtained from Dow Corning that included concerns over implant problems that had not been made public. The jury was persuaded that Dow Corning was at fault and gave Ms. Hopkins $7.3 million.

The story garnered headlines and compounded the pressure brought on the FDA by Weiss, talk shows, and the press. The scientific advisory panel was reconvened in February 1992. The panel heard testimony from plastic surgeons, rheumatologists, and women with implants. They received 30,000 pages of documents describing Dow's safety research. The panel found Dow's evidence insufficient and recommended restrictions on the use of implants.

Meanwhile, Dow Corning had come under public attack for the revelations in the Hopkins trial. Dow made complete public disclosure of all its internal documents. The media reported excerpts from the documents focusing on customer complaints and formerly unreported experimental results. After an unsuccessful damage control effort explained in chapter 8, the company capitulated, withdrew from the implant market, and changed top management.

In April 1992, the FDA ruled that silicone gel breast implants could not be used for augmentation for cosmetic reasons. They could still be used postmastectomy for breast restoration or to replace ruptured or leaking implants. A plan for long-term study was included in the ruling. In effect, the silicone breast implant era was over. Implants might still be obtained, but saline, not silicone, would be chosen.

Throughout this period the medical community, particularly the plastic surgeons, attempted to focus attention on other aspects of the issue. They argued that, because there was no evidence of danger and because so many women had received implants over so many years, it was foolish to be swayed by the hysteria of a few. They talked about the need for scientific study, not anecdotal evidence. They aligned themselves with the manufacturers, but with the collapse of Dow Corning's position, that proved a disastrous strategy. Much of their argument was based on the fact that the vast majority of women with implants were happy with them, referring to a study by Iverson (1991).

Iverson reported that 65% of respondents had implants for augmentation, and the remainder for reconstruction following mastectomy. The three most common reasons were for a more proportionate build (93%), a more appealing appearance (83%), and a boost in self-confidence (76%). Ninety-five percent said their bodies did look more proportional, 90% that they looked more appealing, and 81% that they felt more confident. Ninety-five percent were satisfied with the outcome of their surgery. The 35% who had implants for reconstruction after mastectomy gave as reasons: to be freed from the need to wear an external prosthesis (90%), to help them forget about the state of their health (79%), and to feel "whole again" (75%). Ninety percent agreed that they were freed of the need for the external prosthesis, 80% said that implants helped them forget about the state of their health, and 77% said implants restored a feeling of wholeness. Eighty-nine percent were satisfied with their outcomes. Across both groups, 93% were satisfied and 96% would have the surgery again.

The most frequent side effects mentioned by Iverson were change in nipple sensitivity, increased or decreased, by 40% of the augmentation patients, and hard or moderately firm breasts by 15% of augmentation patients and 26% of reconstruction patients.

When the FDA ruled that implants should be restricted, the country's leading medical journal, the *New England Journal of Medicine*, editorialized that women were now denied the freedom to choose and consent to a procedure they might want. They were being denied the right to informed consent (Angell, 1992). Making medical decisions not based on science was decried (Fisher, 1992). A year later the American Medical Association (AMA) called for the return of silicone implants to the market.

The AMA argument and FDA Chairman David Kessler's response are very interesting to former argumentation teachers like us. What is clearly being debated is where the presumption should rest in the controversy. The AMA said that, because no danger has been proved, implants should be available (Council on Scientific Affairs, 1993). Kessler argued that, because safety had not been proved, they should be banned (Kessler, Merkatz, & Shapiro, 1993). Each sought to place the burden of proof on the other. Under Kessler's leadership the federal government established a national health policy on implants that conflicts with the recommendation of the largest organized medical groups in the nation.

This brief history does not tell the story of how a crucial scientific study guided national health policy. As subsequent chapters reveal, everyone agreed that there was no convincing, careful, scientific study establishing that implants were either dangerous or safe. This was not a health issue decided on clear scientific evidence. The aforementioned history does not tell the story of what was happening within the medical community, or of the conflict between physicians of different specialties. Nor does it reveal the impact of all this public debate on the 2 million women who had implants in their bodies. The chapters that follow attempt to present those stories.

THE TAMPA BAY AREA

One reason we became involved in this project was that the Tampa Bay area, where we lived, and the University of South Florida College of Medicine, where we worked, were important in this controversy. A rheumatologist colleague had been one of the first doctors to speak out saying that silicone might lead to connective tissue disease. Patients came from across the country to see him and his fellow rheumatologists. Because he had testified in implant-related court cases, and before Congress and the FDA, the rheumatologist was known to plaintiffs' attorneys who sometimes suggested that their patients visit him. The legal connection generated criticism from other physicians.

We have already mentioned the role of our plastic surgery colleagues. They had begun research to see if the symptoms being blamed on implants were more often present in women with silicone implants than in women with other kinds of plastic surgery. They were joined shortly after we began our research by a new colleague who was a member of the FDA scientific advisory committee. Community plastic surgeons in Tampa Bay were particularly outspoken in resentment of what the rhuematologists were saying. It is the only case we know of where a formal complaint was filed on this issue by one group of doctors about another. Professional solidarity cracked.

Women in the Tampa Bay Area concerned about the safety of their implants were quite outspoken. They had been featured in some of the early national TV coverage, they were visible in the local press, and they willingly accepted the title Silicone Sisters for their support groups. They frequently wrote letters to the newspaper editors and contacted the reporters who wrote on the topic to make sure their stories were heard. Key players were in our community, the local press coverage was especially intense, and women came from all over the country to see physicians involved. We found ourselves surrounded by this topic.

As we reflect on the research we performed, with the luxury of the time delay the process of writing a book requires, some additional events have occurred. The manufacturers of implants, including Bristol-Meyers Squibb, Dow Corning, Baxter Healthcare, and Minnesota Mining and Manufacturing, have reached a $4.25 billion settlement of a class action suit against them. The number of women who have joined that suit is larger than originally anticipated, reaching 400,000 by May 1995 (Kolata, 1995). Some women joined the suit in response to newspaper ads by attorneys promising compensation even if the women were not currently having problems with their health or implants. As a result, the amount of compensation paid to any one individual is likely to be modest. However, the settlement may be delayed or, perhaps, never be paid at all. On May 15, 1995, Dow Corning, which was to have provided the largest share of the settlement, filed for bankruptcy claiming, "it could not afford to both contribute $2 billion to a breast implant settlement fund and defend itself against independent product liability claims" (Kristof, 1995, p. C7). Judicial determination of that case must precede any payment to the plaintiffs in the class action suit.

Ironically, on the same day that our local newspaper contained an advertisement seeking women who believed they should share in these funds, it also carried a story about a large study done by the Mayo Clinic showing no greater presence of the rheumatological symptoms in women with implants than those without (Gabriel et al., 1994). Among the earliest and most frequent illnesses attributed to silicone gel implant leakage in case descriptions were rheumatological symptoms like scleroderma and arthritis. A substantial body of research is accumulating, which offers reassurance of implant safety. Our plastic surgeon colleagues have published results showing that these symptoms have not appeared more often in women with breast implants than in women who have undergone nose jobs, face lifts, tummy tucks, and the like (Wells, K. E., et al., 1994). Dr. Anthony Watson reported to British Association of Plastic Surgeons that among more than 600 women, those with silicone gel breast implants had no more cases of cancer or connective tissue disease than those without implants ("Support," 1994). Peter Brooks, an Australian rheumatologist, wrote, "There is an increasing body of evidence that suggests that silicone implantation is not associated with significant disease . . ." (1995, p. 433). Fisher claimed that 13 recent epidemiological studies found no link between silicone implants and disease. In presenting their findings of a 14-year study of the more than 87,000 women in the Nurses Health Study cohort, the authors cited 10 studies, all but one since 1992, with similar results: no connection between implants and connective tissue disease (Sanchez–Guerrero et al., 1995). These findings should be reassuring to women with implants and to those considering them. These epidemiological studies, not present early in the controversy, now show the symptoms that first caused concern do not appear to be linked to silicone implants.

On the other hand, the largest study to date (Hennekens et al., 1996) surveyed 395,543 women and found a "small but statistically significant risk" of experiencing some connective tissue diseases among women with breast implants (p. 621). In addition, case reports continue to appear describing women with implants who are ill. Lu, Shoaib, and Patten (1994) concluded that silicone breast implants could be the cause of chest pain from inflammatory reactions and neuromas in 11 women they studied. Spiers, Grotting, and Omura (1994) reported a case study in which a patient's red skin rash and ulceration disappeared following the removal of her silicone implant. Wells, Daniels, Gunasekaran, and Wells (1994) found increased local immune reaction and cellular inflammation in breast biopsies of women with silicone implants when compared with a control group. Yoshida, Teuber, German, and Gershwin (1994) provided a theoretical explanation of how silicone might initiate such inflammatory response and autoreactivity.

Although the large epidemiological studies conducted so far have found no "large risks of connective tissue diseases following breast implants" (Hennekens et al., 1996, p. 616), further research is being conducted to support more definitive conclusions. Moreover, more ambiguous and subjective symptoms reported by women with silicone implants have not been included in the large studies. When the studies showing no relationship between silicone implants and connective tissue disease began to appear, we asked one of our rheumatologist colleagues about them. He replied that he was no longer concerned about silicone causing connective tissue diseases, but was now concerned that the implants caused chronic fatigue syndrome. As we explain in later chapters, patients attributing illness to their implants reported a large number of symptoms in patterns like chronic fatigue or Gulf War syndrome. These do not fit the typical disease templates used by most physicians. Continued concern about silicone implants is associated with complaints that do not fit medicine's usual method of diagnosis. As a result, uncertainty about the relationship between silicone and these ailments persists. And we are mindful that the emerging consensus on leaks and ruptures points to a higher rate of complications than were acknowledged by implant manufacturers before this controversy became public. A recent magnetic-resonance-imaging study found that 10–12 years after implant surgery 91% of the polyurethane-coated implants and 31% of the conventional silicone implants had ruptured (Burton, 1996, p. B4).

The scientific jury is still out on the side effects of silicone implants. Just as clearly, the legal and regulatory juries are in. Whatever the scientific conclusion about the safety and complications of silicone breast implants, it will be late in influencing government policy, the success of silicone gel implant manufacturers, the class action suit settlement, or the opportunity of women to select silicone implants. Plastic surgeons are chastened and rebuilding their image. Reporters have gone on to new controversies. But millions of women still have implants. Perhaps the current news about rheumatological illnesses will offer some comfort to the vast majority of women who feel well. For those who are ill, the uncertainties remain.

What follows are the stories of those involved in the controversy and its impact on the public. They are stories of individuals and institutions searching to understand physical illness, medical risks, and ethical responsibility, at a time when scientific data were inadequate. The accounts tell us much about how patients, physicians, and the public deal with uncertainty. We invite you to share in the ways these stories unfolded to us.

2

STORIES OF IMPLANTS
AND ILLNESS:
LOSS AND CONFUSION

COLLECTING THE STORIES

From summer of 1991 through spring of 1994, we interviewed 35 women who had undergone the breast implant procedure. Twenty of those had sought medical help based on their perception that the implants had caused them health problems. We found those women through the cooperation of local Tampa Bay plastic surgeons and the University of South Florida rheumatology clinic. Interviews with 15 women who were happy with their implants were obtained through the cooperation of local plastic surgeons, volunteers who attended lectures in which initial results of our study were presented, and by word of mouth from women we had interviewed or who had heard about our work. We met with the women in their homes, in plastic surgeons' offices, in a laboratory room of the University rheumatology clinic, in the courtyard of a local hospital, and by the swimming pool of a suburban Holiday Inn. Conversations lasted from 30 minutes to 2 hours and were tape recorded and transcribed.

We used an open-ended, unstructured interview schedule, encouraging women to discuss issues related to breast implants and health that they thought were important. In our interviews, we attempted to minimize our influence, though we recognize that it could not be removed. We encouraged the women to speak at length, using probes and invitations to elaborate. We followed unanticipated topics that the women introduced.

Our desire for an open-ended structure was balanced by the need to cover topics we believed to be central to the controversy: sources of information about implants, individuals involved in the women's decisionmaking, the effect of the implants on self-concept, and interactions with physicians and other health-care professionals. If these topics did not arise in the women's accounts, we asked open-ended questions about them. Although the interviews followed the women's lead, they usually included questions like those developed in the interview schedules in Fig. 2.1 and Fig. 2.2.

1. Tell me the story of what has brought you to where you are now with your implants.
   a. When did you first get implants?
   b. How did you find out about them?
   c. How did you make the decision to have implants?
   d. What did you know about them at that time?
   e. Who did you talk to about getting implants?
   f. What did your doctor say about the implants? Appearance? Side effects/risk? Process of implantation?
   g. What were your expectations about the implants? Appearance? Comfort? Self-esteem?
   h. Were these expectations met?
   i. Who influenced your decision to have the implants?
   j. Who had the most influence?
   k. What kind of implants do you have?
   l. How were they implanted? Under the muscle? On top?
2. How did you feel about that decision right after you had them?
3. How do you feel about it now?
4. Has your level of satisfaction changed?
   a. If changed, when?
   b. What led to the change in your feelings?
5. How have your implants affected your image of yourself?
6. How have they affected your relationship with your spouse or significant others?
7. Do you think your implants have affected your health?
   a. If yes, what makes you say that?
   b. What symptoms, if any, are you having?
   c. When did they begin?
   d. When did you first believe that your implants were making you sick?
8. What do you understand is the relationship between your implants and your health generally?
9. Where have you gotten information about that?
   a. Media?
   b. Friends?
   c. Family?
   d. Doctor?
10. How easy was it for you to get information about this?
   a. In the medical community?
   b. In the media?
   c. Is the information you received consistent?
   d. How have you resolved any contradictions?

FIG. 2.1. Interview schedule for women associating health problems with their implants (continued on next page).

11. When did you first hear the term:
    a. Silicone disease?
    b. Connective tissue disease?
    c. Human adjuvant disease?
12. What do those terms mean to you?
13. Where did you first hear about those diseases?
14. Where else have you gotten information about the disease?
15. What are the possible side effects of the implants?
16. How likely do you think women are to have this kind of response to implants?
17. How do you understand what is happening to your body as a result of the implants(s)?
18. Have you considered having your implant(s) removed?
    a. If yes, what are you thinking about that? Why?
    b. What has led you to consider that?
    c. Who have you talked with about that decision?
    d. How do you feel about the information you are getting?
         1.) Is it consistent?
         2.) Who do you believe more? Why?
19. How do you think removal of your implants would affect your health?
    a. How long might that take?
    b. What side effects might you expect?
20. How do you expect to look if the implants are removed?
21. How would that be for you?
22. Would you consider having a different kind of implant or reconstruction done?
22. Do you know other people who have implants?
    a. If yes, have their experiences with their implants been similar to yours?
23. Have you heard anything about implants on television or in the newspapers lately?
    a. What stories have you read about or seen?
    b. What do you think about those stories?
24. Are there problems related to your implants and your health that you have not had the chance to talk about or questions you have not had answered to your satisfaction? If yes, what are they?
25. Who would you most like to talk to about them?
26. Is there anything we haven't talked about in the interview that you'd like to add or ask?

FIG. 2.1. (continued).

1. Tell me about how you decided to have implants.
   a. When did you first get implants?
   b. How did you find out about them?
   c. How did you make the decision to have implants?
   d. What did you know about them at that time?
   e. Who did you talk to about getting implants?
   f. What did your doctor say about the implants? Appearance?
      Side effects/risk? Process of implantation?
   g. What were your expectations about the implants? Appearance?
      Comfort? Self-esteem?
   h. Were these expectations met?
   i. Who influenced your decision to have the implants?
   j. Who had the most influence?
   k. What kind of implants do you have?
   l. How were they implanted? Under the muscle? On top?
2. How did you feel about that decision right after you had them?
3. How do you feel about it now?
4. Has your level of satisfaction changed?
   a. If changed, when?
   b. What led to the change in your feelings?
5. How have your implants affected your image of yourself?
6. How have they affected your relationship with your spouse or significant others?
7. Do you think your implants have affected your health?
8. Do you know other people who have implants?
   a. If yes, have their experiences with their implants been similar to yours?
9. Have you heard anything about implants on television or in the newspapers lately?
   a. If yes, what stories have you read about or seen?
   b. What do you think about those stories?
   c. If the stories relate to illness, do you think it's likely that women with implants will have these illnesses? Why?
   d. If the stories relate to the FDA or manufacturer's actions, what do you think about the actions these agencies are taking?
10. Is there anything we haven't talked about in the interview that you'd like to add or ask?

FIG. 2.2. Interview Schedule for women not reporting health problems
with their implants.

As is apparent from the length of the interview schedules, the women who believed that their implants had made them ill had more to talk about than the women who did not feel that their implants created problems. Not surprisingly, the length of the interviews differed accordingly.

The object of the interviews was to see the breast implant controversy through the patient's perspective. We attempted to learn how women created meaning out of their health experiences, their interactions with the medical community, the media accounts related to their implants, and their interactions with other women who had implants. We recognize that multiple readings of the women's stories are possible.

In this study, we employed a thematic narrative analysis of the transcripts, similar to that used by Crawford (1984) in his research on the meaning of health. We read the interviews and categorized topics, searching for "integrating concepts." We did not come to the interviews with a theory to test or a hypothesis in place, though there were obviously topics about which we were particularly curious. We did not know what we would find. What follows is a summary of the stories that emerged from our attempt to find the meaning our interviewees were assigning to their experiences.

THE NARRATIVE PERSPECTIVE

The Narrative Idea

We used Fisher's (1984) definition of narration as the basis for our analysis. According to Fisher, narratives are "words and/or deeds—that have sequence and meaning for those who live, create or interpret them" (p. 2). The narrative perspective was helpful for several reasons: a) Narratives are useful for reflecting on the ethical basis of medical decisions. The ethical issues surrounding breast augmentation and implant removal were pervasive in the discussions we had with women and their doctors. b) Personal accounts are helpful when trying to understand the storyteller's sense of identity. c) As sense-making accounts, stories serve as important reasons for the decisions individuals make in their lives, including decisions about their health.

The usefulness of narrative in prompting reflection about medical ethics has been well established (Smith, 1993). Brown (1993) outlined the use of stories and dramatic vignettes "to provide caregivers and ethicists with a resource for . . . moral reflection and creative expression about ethical dilemmas in health care" (p. 3). She credited the use of narrative for "teaching and doing ethics" with its ability to provide a "theoretical home for our appreciation of the tangled swirl of emotions, relationships, power dynamics, diversions, resources, bureaucratic constraints, and happenstance in ethical decision making" (p. 3). Such contextualization often falls outside the boundaries of traditional moral analysis (Smith, 1993).

The ability of narrative analysis to place medical decisions within a context is critical. Holmes (1989) argued that medical decisionmaking is only ethical if it recognizes the situation and context in which patients make decisions and "recognizes their place in relationships that are vital parts of [patients'] lives" (p. 155). Fasching (1989) explained that narrative is "superior to purely theoretical reflection" as a basis for ethical inquiry because it "reflects the complexity, drama, and subtleties of life in its concrete particularities in a way that theoretical reflection cannot" (p. 2). By examining the stories women tell about their experiences with breast implants, we gained insight into the multiple influences which informed their decision making. Such understanding enriches the base of ethical considerations in the practice of medicine.

Narratives also provide us with clues about how individuals create meaning in the midst of confusion. The breast implant controversy has presented difficulty for women and physicians making decisions about health care. The news media, FDA hearings, and courtrooms have been forums for contradictory messages about safety and efficacy. In the throes of conflicting advice and experiences, women use narratives to make sense of their experience (Young, 1990). Women express the sense they have made as they tell about that experience. Stories tell us how random facts and events are ordered and given significance by the storyteller, "The unfolding drama of life is revealed more by the telling than by the actual events told. . . . Stories are less about facts and more about meanings" (McAdams, 1993, p. 28).

In addition, many of our interviewees focused on their sense of identity as females and as legitimate interpreters of their own reality. According to Gergen and Gergen (1983), individuals use narratives to reconstruct a sense of self, "The fact that people believe they possess identities fundamentally depends on their capacity to relate fragmentary occurrences across temporal boundaries" (p. 255). Self-concept plays a major role in women's decisions to have implants. Narrative is an appropriate method of analysis for women's stories about their bodies because storytelling reveals keys to self-perception.

Narratives also provide the basis for decisionmaking. In this controversy, stories compete with other narratives to function as good reasons for medical decisions (Fisher, 1984). Decisions about health are based on the meaning patients give to symptoms and experiences with disease and their physicians. Narratives function to justify decisions already made and determine future decisions (Fisher, 1985). Understanding the narrative themes can help us to understand the basis on which women made decisions about their health. Multiple stories competed for attention within the silicone breast implant controversy. In our interviews with physicians, plastic surgeons advanced a rational account of breast implant safety based on the statistical evidence of efficacy. Several rheumatologists offered case-based physiological accounts of silicone connective tissue disorders. Our examination of women's personal stories about their implants makes public an additional voice for understanding this controversy.

Narrative Analysis

After all the interviews had been transcribed, we focused on the substance of the narratives (Foss, 1989; McAdams, 1993). We looked for the chronology and meaning of events that the women used to shape their experiences. We focused on nuclear episodes that refer to key events in our interviewees' life stories. We also considered the storyteller's characterization of major players, including herself. We focused on the characters' physical and mental traits and how they changed over time. When possible, we noted the emergence of imagoes, "the characters that dominate our life stories. . . . An imago is a personified and idealized concept of the self" (McAdams, 1993, p. 122). Beyond characters and events, we considered the setting of narratives, the circumstances that surrounded events and people. When we considered plot, we focused upon temporal relationships, the way storytellers sequenced events and created causal relationships.

Having examined individual stories, we looked at major themes of the narratives, a "recurrent pattern of human intention. . . . the level of story concerned with what the characters in the narrative want and how they pursue their objectives over time" (McAdams, 1993, p. 67). From these we fashioned collective accounts which represented dominant characters, plots, and settings.

In the remainder of this chapter and the two chapters that follow, we have recreated the stories of women who have implants—those who attribute illness to their implants and those who do not. We tell the stories as collective narratives, attempting to maintain the uniqueness of individual experience while presenting the integrating concepts, or common themes, that unite each group of women. Not all of the women we interviewed shared each experience told in the collective narratives. The themes represented in these chapters represent only the most dominant stories emerging from our analysis.

The accounts of women who believe their implants cause health problems include a dramatic shift occurring when illnesses are associated with silicone. As a result, their stories are divided between two chapters, prediagnosis and postdiagnosis. Prediagnosis narratives are told in the following section. Postdiagnosis stories are related in chapter 3. The stories from women who are satisfied with their implants are told in chapter 4. All the interviewees' names used in our narratives are fictitious, but their stories are real.

PREDIAGNOSIS NARRATIVES: LOSS AND CONFUSION

The women's stories were as different as the sick women themselves. Donna received her first set of breast implants 30 years ago. Nancy had hers for only 2 years. Leslie underwent four different implant surgeries. Yet all 20 women, no matter how different—survivors of breast cancer, deformities, and low self-esteem—shared a common fear. They believed they faced a malady as grave, if not more dangerous, than the cancer or social stigma they hoped breast implants would erase. Chronically ill for as long as 15 years, the women had searched for an explanation for fatigue, unexplained pain, enduring fevers, and skin disease. They all eventually linked their ailments to their silicone breast implants.

Two major themes emerged from the women's prediagnosis stories. They described, (a) the multiple losses associated with the disease, and (b) the frustrating and confusing search for relief.

Illness as Loss

Sick women's narratives are filled with sadness, grief, and sometimes anger about the multiple ways in which their lives have been diminished by breast implant-related problems. Helen's story is a good example of the pervasive changes she believes have been caused by silicone connective tissues disorder. On the day of the interview, Helen was impeccably dressed, coiffed, and made up. She is a quiet, dignified woman. She appeared to be in her late 30s. It was a surprise when she said she was almost 50 years old.

> Marsha: When you told me you were 49 I couldn't believe it.

> Helen: Well, it's because I haven't been living (laughter). Thank, well thank you, that's good, that's good to hear, but, but if I look younger than my age at all I think it's because I've lived such a cloistered life because I just didn't have the energy to [live].

Eighteen years ago Helen had bilateral implants to balance her breasts, which were different sizes, and to remove an extra nipple beneath her right breast.

> Helen: Within months I was sick. I was unable to pick up my toothbrush in the morning, I had extreme exhaustion, I became allergic to all the normal foods that I eat. . . . [I] became chemically sensitive to car exhaust, perfume, chemicals, all of these years since 1976. I can't shop in stores anymore, I get sick. I usually always get sick when I go out into traffic, even, almost immediately, even getting in my car. I can't buy a new car because I can't tolerate the chemicals inside the car. . . . I'm so sick . . . for 15 years I've been sick, constantly sick all the time.

Like Helen, most women linking health problems to their implants do not focus on individual symptoms or discrete diseases. Their stories of illness are global. What stands out are not the specific, individual symptoms of a particular disease, but the holistic, systemic unraveling of the patient's life. According to Nancy, "The problems I have had . . . have affected my life medically, financially, and physically." The implants affected the women's ability to work, relate to others, fulfill family roles, and maintain independence. As Jill put it, "My life is just turned upside down."

The pervasive effects of the illness are conveyed in the before–after frame characteristic of the women's stories. They compare active, full lives before the implants to a significantly diminished existence following the procedure. Their lives are limited in multiple ways: the physical activities they were able to perform, the social roles they fulfilled, the careers they hoped to pursue, the image they held about their bodies, and their sense of themselves as females.

Loss of Physical Strength and Endurance. Many interviewees described themselves as formerly strong women, of uncommon endurance and energy. Following their implants, the women's physical capabilities dramatically decreased. Barbara is typical:

> I built my house. I laid the block. I put the roof on. . . . That's the kind of stuff I do on a normal routine, I mean, I worked three jobs, went to school, took care of the kids . . . everything, and when you go from that to not being able to lift your head up off the pillow, you think . . . I can't do anything [now]. I went Christmas shopping yesterday. A friend of mine drove me out because I don't even feel like driving a lot . . . all we did was go to Target and then we went to Wal Mart . . . we weren't gone 2 hours. I was exhausted. I couldn't pick up my arms . . . I was just like a puppet sitting there. I couldn't do anything.

Like Barbara, many of the storytellers characterized themselves before the implants as active, priding themselves on their physical endurance and strength. As an abused wife, Barbara described herself as a "strong" person, a "rogue." To support her characterization, she ruefully recalled her response to her husband's attacks, "I didn't sit in the corner and get beat on, I mean, I'd knock him down." Jean described herself similarly, "I'm not a pansy." She told us about an incident following surgery when her boss tried to convince Jean to stay at home and recuperate, "He said, 'Damn it, there's no way you can work.' I said, 'Damn it, to hell I can't. I'll show you,' and I did." As she told the story of her defiance, Jean commented on her recently diminished strength, wondering how long she could "drag on before I finally succumb to whatever the hell this is."

The loss of energy was the most common element of the before–after stories. Not all accounts were as developed as Barbara's and Jean's; some comparisons were mere fragments. Leslie "used to go dancing all the time," now she reports, "I was so exhausted mentally and physically [with the illness] I couldn't." Nancy "used to go dancing four, five nights a week" before she became ill. Susan described herself as:

> A very active person, I go up and down ladders, I work on my own houses, you know, I do all, I'm very, very physical, I'm out and about doing these things. I can't step on a ladder now . . . the pain becomes so acute in my feet and legs . . . so I keep them elevated, and even then . . . there are times I can't even move.

Toni concisely summed up the "after" experience of the implants, "You become a couch potato."

Loss of Social Relationships.   Beyond the loss of energy and normal activities that previously characterized their lives, these women also experienced gradual social isolation. As they became more exhausted and less able to participate in daily activities, the storytellers withdrew from family, friends, and romantic-sexual relationships.

Harriet, a former parachutist, avid world traveler, and backpack enthusiast, was confined to a wheelchair during her interview. She described herself before having her implants: "I had strength you wouldn't believe. I [could] get out here and go backpacking with these young people for 3 days in the wilderness at a time . . . and keep right up." Following her implants, she had to give up her athletic pursuits. Along with her activities, she lost her friends: "I said [to my friends], 'Don't you understand, I am never going to climb . . . I can never climb Mt. Baldy again.' See by now I'm on a walker. . . . I watch TV now a little, you know, what else can I do?" Mourning her recent social isolation, Harriet concluded, "This is not just a medical battle, this really reaches into your whole life . . . I lost most of my friends." Because she was unable to join them in their hikes and walks, Harriet's friends finally stopped visiting her.

Unlike Harriet, other women voluntarily withdrew from interaction with significant others. Jean discontinued overnight visits to her mother's home, fearing she would die there, "It's to the point where I was afraid to even spend the night over at my mother's because I didn't want her to wake up and find me dead in her house." Others pushed family and friends away, too exhausted to maintain and nurture relationships: "I was very short with people . . . didn't want to talk to anyone." Karen even limited phone contact, "You don't want to socialize . . . not answer the phone." Toni provided an explanation for social withdrawal; she needed all her energy just to endure. "My mother asked me a question once and I yelled back and said, 'I can't think, just leave me alone.' It's all you can do to survive."

For women with children, the inability to fully perform as parents created the most grief. The illness prevented some women from participating in their children's extracurricular activities and sometimes from fulfilling their roles as protectors and nurturers. Janet was unable to generate sufficient energy and endurance to enjoy her children's performances, "My daughter just turned 9, and my son's 10 . . . I've missed a lot of baseball games . . . I've missed, you know, some dances, and I've missed, I've missed too much." Terry's case was more extreme. Because she lacked energy, her daughter had to become more independent than a 5-year-old should be:

I'll be 31 on Wednesday, my daughter will be 5, we have the same birthday, and we're very close. But I go to bed before her and you know I feel bad, I get her dinner and bathe her and everything and then you know, and she sits up and watches the TV and she goes and turns off all the lights and you know, puts herself to bed. A lot of nights I'm in bed before my own kid is. Yeah, that's pretty bad . . . it's had a bearing on my daughter.

Like Terry, many women described family members as "very supportive," filling in when illnesses overcame family responsibilities. Others, however, reported that their chronic ailments ruptured the family structure. Janet's husband divorced her, "It was too much, you know, I don't blame him [for leaving]." Describing her depression as a "black hole," Janet explained, "I wasn't there for him anymore. And I had always been there for him, and he didn't know how to be there for me." Janet attributed her husband's reaction, in part, to her withdrawal from sexual intimacy. "I wasn't very [intimate with him], I didn't want him close you know." Feeling unwell due to illness and unattractive due to complications of the plastic surgery, Janet didn't feel sexually attractive, and her husband "just couldn't deal with it."

Other women told us about similar withdrawal from physical and sexual contact with men, diminishing their romantic relationships or their hopes for finding one. Unmarried at 45, Jean confided that she had given up her dream of having an intimate relationship. Due to prednisone, a medication prescribed for seizures and potassium problems, she had gained a large amount of weight and developed a hunch back. "Now I have been celibate for . . . many years . . . since I've gotten so you know, grotesque, I feel grotesque. . . . I had hopes of, even at my age, of maybe some day meeting a man and having a relationship." She told us that she had given up hope.

Like Jean, Barbara explained how breast migration and immune system disease had precluded romantic and sexual relationships with men. Reluctant to be seen unclothed, Barbara felt she no longer matched the expectations that men had about good female companionship:

> Who wants to be around a man when you're not, physically feel[ing] well? Number one, you don't feel well, you don't feel good about yourself. [The implants] were ugly; one's up here, one's down here. [The man would say], "Oh yeah, I slept with this girl, she's freaky looking, you know." Nobody wants to deal with that; anybody that sleeps with somebody else has got to feel good about themselves. That age-old story, "you gotta like yourself before anybody else will." Well, I like myself, but I didn't like the way my body looked . . . and I didn't feel good, I don't feel good enough to sleep with anybody, I feel like poop, you know? I mean who wants to be around somebody that feels bad all the time? . . . I mean men like cute, sweet, skinny, upbeat, pleasant, happy-looking people, you know, they never complain, never bitch . . . never groan, you know, that kinda thing and I'm just not that kind of person anymore. . . . I don't feel like getting dressed and going out, looking for men.

Like Barbara, most of the women we talked to had suffered severe social losses, either with friends or family. The cost of the illnesses was measured in people as well as pain.

Career and Financial Loss.   An additional loss for about half the women we interviewed was their careers. The illness, exhaustion, complications, and surgeries took their toll. Women talked about their inability to perform the tasks required for financial independence. Before her implants, Jill used to work two full-time jobs:

I used to work . . . 92½ hours every week. . . . Never bothered me. . . . I worked at a flower shop during the day and I tended bar at night. So I was on my feet constantly, you know, and now, 2 hours, if I have to stand more than 2 hours I'm worthless.

Sarah was also disabled, "I can't go back to work, and . . . we're financially strapped." At the time of the interview, Sarah and her husband were surviving on disability.

For some women, the inability to work represented the loss of a dream and a threat to independence. Helen, a single mother, explained the financial ruin that accompanied her illness:

I'm a professional artist. . . . I had a career going very well when I had the implants put in. I started in 1972 and then I got sick right away at the end of 1976, so my career has been very, very rocky . . . there is a company manufacturing collectible porcelain dolls and figurines from my work, and I have, I have been so sick that I have not even put together a contract, so . . . I mean they can't do this without paying royalties, but the point is that I don't have a contract and I don't have the royalty agreements set, and . . . my career that I had started really came to a halt. I couldn't keep up with, I couldn't think about what is current in the market . . . what's selling, colors. . . . I've really been limping along in that business and having to borrow money. . . . It's been very, very devastating because . . . when I started in business in 1972 and about 1973 I purchased my own home. I've been divorced for 22 years and raised my daughter, but I was able to purchase my own house, and . . . I've almost lost it several times because of the illness.

Financial ruin was only part of the loss. Diminished career opportunities caused some women to wonder about the quality of their lives after implants. Donna invested herself in her career. With her ability to work threatened, she explained how futile her future appeared: "I think the thing that frightens me the most is I have another 25 years to work and what if I'm not able to work? Working was my whole life. I mean, I think that we all have to do something where we feel that we are needed."

The Diminished Body Image: Loss of Self-Esteem. Beyond the loss of relationships and work, some women's stories described a diminished body image. Although many women were happy with the appearance of their implants, other stories included disappointment and chronic aesthetic problems: encapsulation (hardening), migration, and/or granulomas. By the time we interviewed the patients, many had undergone multiple plastic surgeries, replacements due to ruptures, capsular contraction, and leakage. For these women, the aesthetic results they hoped for had either not been realized or had caused side effects that were physically disfiguring. Janet described her implant surgery as "a mess. . . . The implants were way up high in the chest wall, the sutures around the nipples were . . . very sloppy . . . there was puckering." Susan described her implants as "misshapen." For Janet, and several others, breast migration was common, "The implants were migrating; one went way up high in the chest wall and the other went underneath my arm." Nancy's implant had moved, "sliding back under my arm pit . . . I had to pull it forward in order to put my arm down." Barbara described a similar problem with the positioning of one set of implants:

> The one implant had pulled itself up and capsulated and was up here . . . it was up here in a knot and it was literally ripping the muscles off the wall of my chest, and you could see . . . indentures in my side where the muscles were just being ripped and tore up my body.

Some migration took the form of granulomas, migrating pieces of silicone that broke away from the implants forming masses in the body. Carol, a young woman who was grateful for the increased self-esteem that breast implants had given her, told us about the longitudinal masses that had formed inside her arms. Surgery to remove the masses had cut into her muscle tissue. She explained that the surgeon had to make incisions beneath the breast and "underneath my arm to clean, to clean all this out. He cut away quite a bit of tissue . . . and said he could not get all the silicone out." Carol showed us the thick pink scars that lined the underside of her arms. She worried about the scars left by the removal of the silicone: "It's still pretty fresh, hopefully it'll get better, but he did have to cut away some of the muscle."

Some of the women had undergone several procedures for removing leaks and ruptures, leaving their chests scarred and misshapen. For some the results caused shame and diminished body image. Janet reported, "I'd cry every time I took a shower, I couldn't stand looking at myself." Susan told us that she avoided looking directly at her implants. For women who originally had implants to improve their appearance, many felt "betrayed" and "angry" that they had been misled about the outcome of their surgery. Harriet explained:

> I was very angry because prior to the operation [the surgeon] had taken me in a special room and showed me photographs, pictures of these beautiful women and said he had done those . . . and I came out hideous. . . . [He] led me to believe that I would come outa' there like a movie star; didn't wanna' be a movie star but wanted my dress to fit me better.

Harriet, like many of the women we talked to, regretted her decision to have implants: "I should have stayed with just letting it be."

Loss of Gender.   Most of these women had their implants permanently removed or were planning removal. Having originally chosen implants to feel more womanly, they now faced the choice of losing their breasts. Although the decision to remove the implants usually came after diagnosis of silicone tissue disorder, the narrative theme is included here because it reinforces the experience of loss so characteristic of the illness stories.

During a group interview with five women from Denver, Toni explained the multiple complications that had led her to finally have her implants removed. Dressed in loose clothing that concealed the form of her body, she also had a short, boyish hair cut. Angry, she loudly declared to the group, "Okay, I'll show you. This is what I can live with for the rest of my life. Isn't that wonderful?" She pulled her baggy top over her and stood in front of us revealing a chest that was a maze of red scar tissue. Concave indentions replaced her breasts. She had no nipples or roundness indicating where breasts should have been. Marsha explained her own reaction to what she saw: "I instinctively crossed my arms across my breasts, as if to protect them from similar mutilation. My reaction gave me visceral proof that the loss of the implant represented more than the removal of a medical device, but a loss of part of one's self." Karen's explanation of her own decision confirmed this interpretation:

I had, you know, one mastectomy and then a little while later I had the other one removed, now I can have both of them removed again? . . . even though they're implants, and they're, they become part of your body. . . . I mean these feel like they're my breasts even though I know that they're implants. And so what every single person in here went through was, was losing a part of yourself. . . . It has a lot to do with your self-esteem . . . your femininity, you know.

For many women interviewed, breasts (including implants) represented womanhood itself. And the loss of the implants equaled the loss of femininity. One woman explained that as a result of losing both breasts and implants, "I've lost my gender. I don't have it any more. I don't have any gender." Toni, augmented as a result of sagging breasts due to nursing, explained that she felt neutered upon the removal of her implants:

I gave all my dresses away, I, I can never find anything that looks [good] on me like a skirt or a dress, so I wear sloppy old sweats or tennis clothes and go play tennis, or I'm, I'm not male gendering it up but I've lost my gender, I've, I've lost it and you can say "well, it's that just because you don't have bumps on your chest." Well if you wanted to say that's a part of it, yeah, that's a part of it. But I think that's too simple.

The loss of femininity created feelings of inadequacy for some women. Stripped of her gender, Sarah felt ashamed and abnormal, "I felt like a freak, without anything in me."

With a diminished sense of self and a decreased ability to enjoy friends, family, work, and leisure, women with implant problems were described as "the crushed and broken pieces." The all-consuming nature of the illness they associated with their breast implants emerged repeatedly in these narratives. The stories are heart rending. Toni explained the impact of the disease on members of her implant support group: "We are all caught up in this earth-shaking situation, life-destroying situation." She described silicone connective tissue disease as "a psychological trauma of the worse sort."

The first overarching theme we found in these women's stories was illness as loss. Diminished lives were described as loss of physical strength and endurance, loss of social relationships, loss of career and financial opportunity, loss of self-esteem, and loss of gender. Our interviewees described their lives as having lost vital elements. Their stories were moving as we heard them and continue to touch us as we reread and remember them. No matter what one's view of the silicone gel breast implant controversy, its causes, the role of media, manufacturers, government, and doctors, or the scientific facts, one cannot escape appreciating that these women have seen their lives changed in tragic ways. Any discussion that ignores or diminishes the pain and distress they experienced misses a central fact, perhaps the most central fact, of the controversy. It is no surprise that stories like those we were told made compelling news and influenced the regulators who heard them. It could not have been otherwise

The Frustrating Search for Diagnosis and Relief

If each of us strives earnestly to author a meaningful narrative of our experience, how much more intense must have been the struggle for coherent meaning by these women whose losses were so severe? Underlying the diminished lives they described were multiple unexplained symptoms and a series of unsatisfactory meetings with physicians as they sought to understand and alleviate illness. Melanie's story highlights the confusion and futility of the search that characterized many accounts:

> I started having problems a few weeks after that with the implants, I got a big infection in 'em and everything, and since then it's just been like a down hill battle with 'em, it's always been one thing after another. . . . The implants were placed directly in, and then 3 weeks after that I had an infection in where the skin turned real black . . . I mean problem after problem with them and I kept getting infections and they, they became encapsulated and that's when I had another operation to remove the one's that were in there. I've had three sets . . . And there was a bunch of lymph nodes . . . they just kept swelling up . . . the right one [breast] I have drainage in; this left side is just completely numb . . . swelling of the joints and dryness in your eyes, your mouth . . . I've had a rash that would come up on my hands and my feet . . . my dermatologist didn't know where it was coming from . . . they had me on prednisone by mouth and it was like making me sick.

> Since all this started with the implants, I get colds easier and infections, like these little skin cancers they've been freezing off for a little over a year now, they just keep coming back. Nothing heals, I mean, every time I turn around they have to put me on antibiotics to get anything to heal. And the swelling. . . . I had swelling in my hand and in the wrist, my knee and my ankle. My menstrual cycle . . . has been irregular for a little over a year now, and I don't know if that's anything to do with it.

Melanie's story is typical of many women who blame illnesses on their breast implants. Following a rupture or leak (recognized only months or years after the breakage), multiple, unexplainable, seemingly unrelated illnesses befall the storyteller. The symptoms linked to implants ranged from freezing sensations to feelings of being burned with a cigarette. Almost all reported chronic, debilitating fatigue. In all, women described over 80 symptoms.

The symptoms fall into 14 rough groupings. Skin problems were among the most commonly reported afflictions: scleroderma, dermatomycistis, skin cancers, rash, numbness, intense itching, and inexplicable bruising. Lung diseases were also frequently reported: bronchitis, collapsed lungs, breathing difficulties, burning lungs, shortness of breath, chronic choking, and constant colds. Many of the women's illnesses were related to chronic fevers or irregularities in body temperature including chills, burning, and profuse sweating. Women also described aches and pains: headaches, migraines, joint pains, tennis elbow, arthritis, aching breasts, thoracic pain, and chest pain. Complications from surgery were common: fluid in the breast cavity, open wounds, staph infection, and major bleeding. Some women described urinary tract problems: bladder problems, bladder surgery, an inability to urinate, kidney problems, clastic bladder, and odorous urine. Reproductive problems were also linked to implants: hysterectomies, irregular menstrual cycles, "female problems," and ovary removal. Some women had problems with their limbs: the inability to stand, walk, or move without pain; difficulty lifting or stretching arms; unexplainable broken bones; and discolored hands and legs. Digestive problems included nausea, diarrhea, potassium loss, weight loss, and weight gain. Some women experienced swelling in their lymph nodes, breasts, hands, feet, knees, and ankles. Several women labeled their illnesses "immune system problems" or autoimmune disease including high white cell count and an inability to heal. A variety of miscellaneous symptoms were also related to the implants: allergies, sinus problems, dizzy spells, crest syndrome, cancer, dry eyes and mouth, seizures, and chronic flu symptoms. Beyond physical symptoms, mental problems were also included in the women's accounts of their illness: disorientation, memory loss, depression, irritability, impaired concentration, and anxiety. Although most symptoms occurred in locations removed from the breast, women also described aesthetic problems with the implants: encapsulation, seepage, multiple replacements, rupture, migration, granulomas, poor placement, and poor stitching.

On average, the women we talked to each attributed a half dozen symptoms to their breast implants. Like Melanie, the symptoms did not cluster under any one category but were spread across the 14 groupings. Uniting the diverse symptoms was the intensity and mystery of the illnesses. Mary highlighted the severity of her discomfort, calling it the "pain that comes on like an attack . . . [it was so bad] you would actually lose bodily functional control." Women described the symptoms as pervasive and intense, "I have pain in my neck, I have pain in my upper body, I have pain in my fingers that's so bad I can't open an envelope . . . and it seems to be getting worse." Jean suffered from intense burning as well as pain, "I developed hot spots . . . on the arm . . . ankle, my back. . . . and it starts expanding . . . by the time it gets to that half-dollar size, it feels like I've taken a cigarette and just dug in there."

Faced with chronic, pervasive, debilitating symptoms, women tried to find relief. Examples of how women coped with irregular body temperature demonstrate their futile efforts. Jill could not get cool enough, "My skin's on fire. Standing in the shower doesn't help but in my mind it thinks, 'I'm burning, get something cool on me.'" Helen's strategy was equally unsatisfactory, "I slept in my coat and hat and boots and gloves under electric blankets. I could not get warm." Terry was successful in overcoming chills or burning, only to have her temperature swing to the opposite extreme: "I have been cold since the day I came out of the operating room. . . . It's been . . . a constant battle with the shivers, and then I put the blankets on and then I'm hot, it's you know, hot and cold, hot and cold."

The illness story progressed as a debilitating mystery, the storyteller was unable to determine the origins of the complaints, nor was she able to overcome them. Sarah explained:

> I work in an emergency room in a hospital . . . I was just catching everything that came by to me. I was really sick. I had three viruses in December; everything that came through caught at my resistance . . . I had bronchitis, I had been sick for a long time . . . I didn't know what to lay it to, you know. I never could put my finger on it.

Even in consultation with physicians, the illnesses remained unrelieved and undecipherable. When Jill experienced sharp pain in her arm, she sought professional help, "No one could figure [it] out." She asked doctors, "What's there?" Her physicians couldn't find the source of the pain, "Nothing's there. We don't feel nothing." Women consulted one doctor after another, trying successive treatments. Donna sought help from a series of orthopedic surgeons because she thought that arthritis was causing her pain. Different surgeons prescribed steroids, cortisone, and, finally, physical therapy. At the time of the interview, Donna was still experiencing pain.

Donna's story is typical; almost all of the women visited a series of physicians in an effort to find a successful treatment. Mary counted off the number of physicians she had seen and medicines she had tried: "Over these last 7 months I've seen so many different kinds of doctors, I've got a list of medicines this long. When I have a bad reaction to one they keep switching to something else."

Doctors prescribed multiple tests and performed procedures which failed to diagnose the problem. When trying to determine the cause of an enduring fever, Harriet's doctor ordered:

> Blood test, urine test, this test, that test, all came out showing nothing wrong with me, you know. I kept getting worse . . . I was tired, weak and having all these bladder infections and then I had a bad kidney infection. . . . They gave me every test there is to have. . . . At first [doctors in my community] thought it was flea bites. . . . It's been a long circuitous route since the flea bite diagnosis. . . . I was even checked for having AIDS.

Some doctors made inaccurate diagnoses and sometimes prescribed treatments with grave side effects for the storyteller. Jean's physician:

> came to the conclusion that I had Addison's disease, so they put me on potassium . . . I ballooned . . . I got the hump [hunchback]. And I felt better, but I was thoroughly disgusted . . . I'd always been tiny. . . . I'm very self-conscious about it. Six or seven years later, an endocrinologist did three different tests and they came back inconclusive. He did not feel I had Addison's and that upset me, because I'm lying there and I'm thinking, you know, here I am a blimp and I didn't have to be this way, something else was wrong, but what? . . . My hump has never gone down.

Rather than gaining weight like Jean, Mary lost an organ due to misdiagnosis. Surgeons removed her gall bladder when she had severe chest pain: "Nine months after that surgery the exact same attack came back which shocked the heck out of me." Wondering how she could suffer from a gall bladder that had been removed, the doctors, "did look everywhere else and so far except for a continuing high white cell count they can't explain which other organ is doing it." Mary reported that she had received different diagnoses from three different doctors.

During the process of trying to unravel the illness, women reported being diagnosed and treated for a variety of illnesses including premature aging, leukemia, Epstein–Barr syndrome, low thyroid, Addison's disease, tennis elbow, clastic gall bladder, clastic stomach, clastic bladder, Lyme disease, and fibromyalgia.

Following futile attempts at diagnosis, women became discouraged. Having gone from physician to physician in search of relief, Janet explained the disappointment she felt in physicians when they failed to diagnose her problem or relieve her suffering:

> All these years I've been going "What's wrong with me, what's wrong with me?" . . . I'd find a doctor and he'd say, "I can help you." Then no relief, and then he would lose faith in me and I would lose faith in him, and there I was on to try to find another doctor, and one right after the other.

In their stories, women lost faith in physicians when the doctors dismissed their physical symptoms as imaginary, normal, or psychologically based. The women frequently reported being told that the problem was psychosomatic: "Some doctors look at you like you've lost your mind." Barbara considered forgoing medical treatment because she did not want to be called insane, "I almost didn't come to the appointment because I, I didn't want to come and be told again I'm crazy when I know that I'm sick." Seeking relief from an oncologist, Barbara was diagnosed as depressed, "[He] made me an appointment with the psychiatrist last week . . . because he thinks all my symptoms are psychological . . . [according to him] I'm a classic depression."

Other physicians denied the women's illness experiences completely. Mary recounted her interactions with multiple physicians. Complaining of chronic fatigue, pain, and mental nervousness, the doctors told her, "That's normal." When she complained of being "cold all the time." The doctor replied, "Oh that's normal." She explained: "All these things were supposed to be normal so I kept telling myself there was nothing wrong with me. . . . It's normal that you're now going to bed at 7 o'clock at night. . . . it's normal that you just don't feel good."

Jean's physician diagnosed her swelling breast pain and choking as a lack of sex: "You go through those things and you've got doctors that are saying, 'There's nothing wrong; you need to have more sex, or some sex. That will take care of it all.'" Jean was not convinced. Her voice was filled with sarcasm, and she laughed explaining, "Yeah. That's [sex] going to take care of the headaches, the sweats, the chest . . . "

The sick women's stories center around mysterious and debilitating clusters of illnesses, which appear following their implants. They searched in vain for relief and explanation for their symptoms. Along the way, physicians provided little help and sometimes prescribed procedures with harmful side effects. The women moved from one physician to another, trying different medications and diagnoses without relief. Along the way, some physicians doubted the women's sanity and denied their physical experiences. Women lost faith in those physicians.

IMPLICATIONS OF THE PREDIAGNOSIS NARRATIVES

The Doctor–Patient Relationship

The prediagnosis stories reveal the women's disappointment with their physicians and have important implications for doctor–patient relationships. The importance of good rapport between physicians and their patients has been well established. Successful treatment of disease has been linked to the physician's attitude toward his or her patients, the patient's perception that the doctor is taking her seriously, and the confidence which the patient places in the physician (Cousins, 1979, p. 57). In short, "Patients want doctors who will care about them as well as treat them" (Smith & Pettegrew, 1986, p. 137; Smith & Occhipinti, 1984). The prediagnostic stories reveal a dynamic tension between patients' experiences, which when combined with physicians' diagnostic processes and agendas, have a high potential for damaging the crucial rapport between parties. In addition, the patients' unfulfilled need for explanation appears to play a key role in the loss of faith that the women experienced with their doctors.

Common Diagnostic Practice.   Doctors' tendency to adhere to the "relevance rule" and the differential diagnostic process used by most clinicians conflict with women's experiences of their illness. Young (1989) explained that physicians control the course of a medical interview through the relevance rule "that the discourse stay within the realm of medicine" (p. 157). Anything that is not directly related to a specific symptom is considered irrelevant to the medical interview. In her study of physician–patient interaction, Todd (1989) confirmed Young's theory, stating that doctors displayed "boredom, irritation or both" with women patients who told their "life story" during doctor visits (p. 81). Brody (1987) explained that "overworked and harried physicians display little tolerance for any information from patients that is not already formulated as, or at least easily translated into, the 'standard medical history'" (p. 3).

Yet, the patients' stories suggest that women with implant problems see their illnesses as comprehensive, extending into their work lives, leisure activities, and intimate relationships. Their stories are value-laden and emotional. The women explained their diseases through comparisons of their multiple roles and activities before and after the implants. The devastating effects of the illnesses were described only in part as symptoms. They were often connected to the deeper social, vocational, and personal aspects of the women's identities. As a result, when women tell physicians about their problems, they are likely to "break the frame" of the relevancy rule, moving beyond the topics found on the standard medical history form. The physician, focusing on discrete symptoms, might easily miss the women's experiences, dismissing them as irrelevant. Searching for the objective facts, the physician might well ignore the feelings and emotions so important in the patient's story (Smith & Pettegrew, 1986). The patient could easily interpret the physician's inattention to her priorities, values, relationships, and feelings as disconfirmation. The dynamic clearly has the potential for distancing the physician and the patient. Such a circle of misunderstanding cannot aid in the healing of diseases experienced by the women interviewed.

Compounding the potential for misunderstanding is the approach most physicians use in diagnosing illness. Differential diagnosis, as commonly practiced by clinicians, includes the process of comparing the patient's presenting symptoms to a constellation of symptoms typical of known illnesses: "The key element in diagnosis is . . . 'syndrome recognition': a capacity to re-identify, in fresh cases, a disability, disease, or injury one has encountered (or read about) in earlier instances" (Jonsen & Toulmin, 1988, p. 41).

Differential diagnosis involves the identification of a discrete and limited number of symptoms clustering around a particular illness. It would be unusual for a patient to present a large number of seemingly unrelated complaints and have the physician pronounce a single cause.

The women's stories of illness confound the process of differential diagnosis. They included approximately 80 symptoms that they attributed directly or indirectly to leaking silicone. Such a number of ailments, ranging from shortness of breath to weight loss and burning spots, defies the differential process that typifies medical diagnosis. Patients who present multiple symptoms are a challenge to the process and the time constraints of many physicians. Under such conditions, the potential for irritation and disconfirmation is great.

In addition, the chronic nature of the women's ailments presents a challenge. The narratives include multiple doctor visits, medical tests, and medications that fail to resolve the women's problems. The chronically sick woman presents a challenge to the physician's values of curing and efficacy. Such a violation holds the potential to create discomfort, not only for the patient but also for the physician. In such cases, doctors can react with the desire to avoid contact and withdraw from patients (Vanderford, Smith, & Harris, 1992). As a result, physicians might communicate a desire not to spend time or give attention to patients who seem to be nonresponsive to the doctor's ongoing, best efforts.

Women who break the relevance rule by presenting multiple nonclustering symptoms and who are chronically ill present special challenges for doctors who are pressed for time and are pressured to appear omniscient. The temptation to avoid, ignore, and dismiss such patients can be significant. The loss of faith reported in the sick women's stories might well be the result of the conflict between doctors' agendas and patients' experiences.

Psychosocial Needs and the Search for Meaning

Further division between physicians and patients might be attributed to psychological needs which, according to the women's stories, are not being met by doctors. The relationship between psychosocial conditions and physical health has been well established (Brody, 1987; Cousins, 1979). According to Brody, patients often improve physically when they experience a "positive change in the meaning . . . attach[ed] to the illness experience" (p. 6). One of the critical components required for such change is an explanation of the illness. Describing the importance of diagnosis for patients, Brody characterized the diagnosis as a means of demystfying the experience of illness. Categorizing the illness can create a positive experience by providing a cause for the disruption that the illness creates.

The mystery characterizing the women's search for relief heightens their need for explanation. Having repeatedly visited physicians to find no definable ailment, many women expressed despair and hopelessness. The illness narratives stripped women of the very characteristics, activities, and roles that constituted their preimplant identities. Having lost jobs, social relations, self-esteem, and normal movement, women were vigorously searching for causes to explain the disconnection from their previous lives:

> Affliction . . . is a disordering event in that it implies a deviation from a common universe of experience and a disruption of existing personal relations, activities, and social roles. As a disorienting experience, it requires a cognitive reordering. . . . All healing systems, reflecting underlying cultural paradigms, attempt to account for the apparent disorder and through such accounts·including disease categories, theories of causality, and prescriptions for recovery·reduce the dislocation occasioned by the affliction. By helping the afflicted person to answer the questions, "Why me?" and "Why now?" dominant values and categories for understanding reality . . . are reaffirmed. (Crawford, 1984, pp. 61–62)

Remaining within the medical community, few of the women reported receiving any answers to the questions "Why me?" or "Why now?"

Just as clearly, not just any diagnosis will create positive meaning. The "illness experience must be given an explanation . . . that will be viewed as acceptable, given the patient's existing belief system and worldview" (Brody, 1987, p. 6). In prediagnosis stories, physicians' early diagnoses had not resulted in relief. Later diagnoses of psychological disorder, imaginary ailments, and routine aging did not fit into the patients' existing sense of self. Such explanations did not match the strong, active, and emotionally stable images that women held of themselves. To be told that, without reason, they had become mentally ill or prematurely old did not fit the women's deeply imbedded sense of identity.

Her self-image challenged, the woman was left without the ability to make sense out of her experiences. Narrative theory suggests that such incongruities can create even greater suffering. Illness is compounded by the inability to create a coherent account of one's experience (Brody, 1987).

The women's stories of loss and disconfirmation represent a search for explanation and coherence in the midst of continued pain and diminished lives. At every turn in the prediagnosis accounts, coherence is denied. After countless attempts, no resolution is found, and the very experts who are supposed to help patients understand and resolve their illness are sources of denial. Feeling unheard by physicians and finding no source of meaning in the doctors' diagnoses, the women's faith in their physicians diminished. They eventually placed that trust in other agencies.

STORIES OF IMPLANTS AND ILLNESS: DIAGNOSIS AND DIRECTION

The sick women's stories turn on the point of diagnosis. The prediagnosis accounts in the previous chapter are stories of loss, disorientation, and confusion, but once they made their own diagnoses, the patients' stories changed in tone and direction. The women were able to discover feelings of optimism and hope. Postdiagnosis accounts are narratives of women taking action, often in opposition to their physicians.

THE DIAGNOSIS

I had been sick for a long time, just sick, and . . . I never . . . could put my finger on it. . . . Well, one morning I was, I work 11 to 7 at night . . . and I was cleaning up, getting ready to go home, and all of the newspapers for the different departments come through us because we're there all night, and I saw this article there that Dr. X . . . had written on this problem, a silicone problem, and . . . I just looked at it, and I picked it up and I took home with me. Probably didn't read it for 2 weeks and when I did, I was still sick with bronchitis and it was like my lungs were just collapsing on me, and when I read the article, it was just me. . . . So I called his office and he got me right in the next day. And within 2 weeks they had 'em out, here. And so now, I'm much better.

Having sought diligently and unsuccessfully for a diagnosis through legitimate medical sources, Sarah, and others we talked to were frustrated and confused until they serendipitously found an explanation in an unexpected source. Sarah came across a single newspaper article that changed her life and her beliefs about her illness. Jill's discovery was also an unplanned event. Suffering from fever and chronic fatigue for months, Jill decided her illness was imaginary. A few months later her husband was watching television, "[He] was flipping through the channels on TV and Geraldo Rivera come up. . . . And there was something on there about these implant problems. So he just stopped, you know, knowing what I had and all." As he watched the program, Jill's husband became excited, "and, he just calls me and says, 'you gotta come in here.'" As she watched the program, Jill was amazed, "I'm just sitting watching my whole life on this TV screen, you know."

For more than three fourths of the women we talked to, the news media provided an unexpected connection between their health problems and the silicone implants. The Connie Chung news program, *Face to Face*, broadcast December 10, 1990, and again November 11, 1991, was cited by several women as their first point of discovery (Lack, 1990). Nancy had suffered from numbness in her breast, shoulder, and elbow. She experienced chronic pinching pain underneath the implant. Her husband associated his wife's problems with stories told by women on *Face to Face*, "I saw the second . . . program is when I said to Nancy, you should have seen this program because I thought it was you up there talking about your experiences." Nancy's reaction was surprise, "I had no idea that, that my aches and pains and tiredness and . . . lack of wanting to do things would be related to the implant."

Face to Face proved to be an important turning point for Jean as well, who, hearing from friends that the program had aired, sent for a copy of the transcript, "After I read that I thought, 'Well shit, Jean, now you're . . . a walking toxic waste dump. . . . I thought, Shit, damn, no wonder you're sick.' It explained a lot to me, more than a damn doctor."

Although *Geraldo* and *Face to Face* were the most cited television programs, a variety of news sources were identified as helpful:

> I got my information from a *Reader's Digest* 1991, January article, and when I asked my doctor about it, [he said] "I don't know." . . . I never equated any of it with the implants until just last two months . . . I didn't associate it until I read that *Reader's Digest* article.

Susan found her symptoms reflected in a "two-paragraph article, a tiny, little article in the *Lakeland Ledger* and it addressed the subject of the silicone implants." Paula became concerned about her shortness of breath "after hearing all that I've heard on TV." Another woman reported, "I have it all on tape—*Sally Jesse Raphael, Connie Chung*, and *Geraldo*."

As they watched or read news accounts linking their symptoms to the silicone in their breast implants, the women recalled feeling hopeful and optimistic. Janet read an article about local research on silicone connective tissue disorder. She explained her reaction to the diagnosis:

> I feel fine knowing that . . . I know what's causing me to be so sick. If someone fell down and they'd been sick, really sick and couldn't deal with it anymore and no one knew what was causing it and all of a sudden they found out it was a callus on the bottom of your foot . . . you'd be ecstatic, at least they know . . . what they have to deal with.

Helen's reaction to *Face to Face* was similar. She found not only a reason for her illness, but also for hope: "I mean to hear on the *Connie Chung* show, to um, validate a reason for being sick all of these years, I . . . I felt encouraged that at last I might get well." Janet recalled reading a news article about a local rheumatologist's work, "It's like taking the first step. Now you know. Now you know what you're up against, you know. And now there's hope."

For some women, hope was combined with the assurance that they were not insane. Fearing she was prematurely aging, Terry found comfort in the newspaper, "I . . . started the newspaper and reading . . . everything. I started realizing that, hey, there's something here that's more than just my, my imagination." Reassurance that it was not "all in their minds" came for some women through identification with others suffering the same symptoms. While watching *Geraldo*, Jill exclaimed, "And they're these women describing every single thing I've been going through for these past, like by this time it's like 6, 8 months." When Sarah read about symptoms other implant patients were having, she exclaimed, "It was just me."

MEDIA: CONDUITS FOR GUIDANCE AND CONNECTION

I've seen a lot of shows and have some transcripts from some of the shows like *Geraldo* and *Sally Jesse Raphael*. And I think they have been really good to inform the public, not only the pros but the cons, because there are some pros you know, and I think that they've been really good . . . because every program I've watched they had people for it and against [implants].

Many women, like Sarah, told us that the media provided them with information, guidance, and direction beyond the initial diagnosis. Melanie identified television as a primary source of information available to women, "There was nothing really out for a woman or anybody to read except for what you would see on television and that would be it." Finally, believing they had definitive information about the nature and cause of their ailments, the women used the news media as a basis for making decisions about their health.

Some women measured the progression of their illness and chances of recovery by comparing symptoms to those presented by women in the media accounts:

[The women on these shows] some of them are a little worse than me, and some of them are a little better than me . . . but you can listen . . . to some of them and they'll explain like, they'll start here and this is how it goes. And I'll say, "Oh, I'm at this point, you know, where this woman is, and now she can't even work because she doesn't have no brain left." You know, she's completely lost all of her memory and . . . everything, so I worry you know, but I try not to let . . . you can worry yourself sick.

Mary read multiple news accounts while trying to decide whether to have her implants removed. She remarked, "Every book you pick up now has articles about the silicone problem." She linked her implants to thoracic pain, rashes, and fatigue by reading the news. She concluded, "If there's a chance, that's it [silicone causes the illness], I want to try it."

Having found the media accounts personally informative, women reported taking them to their doctors. Armed with a satchel full of newspaper clippings and video recordings, Jill never visits a physician without the media proof of her silicone illness. She explained, "Doctors are too busy to stay at home and watch these things or read these things. Unless somebody sticks it under their nose a lot of doctors miss it. So, that's what I've been doing." Jill keeps her physician informed about current progress in the controversy by sharing news articles and videotapes with her. During one visit, Jill's female physician revealed that the news had more than professional interest for her. When she took a tape of *Geraldo* to her doctor, the physician responded, "'I don't believe this!' And I said, 'Why?' And she goes, 'I have implants!'" Subsequently the physician used the news to monitor the condition of her own implants.

Having served as the basis for initial diagnosis and understanding of silicone illness, news media also served as a powerful conduit for reaching other sources of help. The women recalled how television, radio, newspapers, and magazines led them to rare sympathetic physicians, attorneys, and support networks. Janet, Nancy, and Terry found their way to a rheumatologist specializing in implant-related illnesses through newspaper articles, "The local paper, yeah. That's when we picked up Dr. X's name." "I read about Dr. X in the newspaper . . . after my biopsies. There was an article on him and his associate, and I . . . the research they were doing." Donna recalled, "I . . . started clipping all the newspaper articles. I found a couple of newspaper articles and I called the physicians that had written the articles."

Other women found direction for financial reparation. Barbara concluded, "If it hadn't been for all the [media] exposure . . . we've had recently about silicone poisoning" her insurance would not have paid for the replacement of her implants. Leslie found her way to an attorney helping women make legal claims based on their illnesses:

> The attorney whose name appeared in the paper, I called him to see if my symptoms, because I had been going to my doc . . . they kept telling me I had fibromyalgia. [He said] "Just do exercise, there's nothing more, just exercise and you'll become well." So the article in the newspaper, named the attorney and he is who I called and I told him my symptoms, and asked him if they were similar to those ladies and he said "Yes."

Media also played a role in creating support systems for women. Television, magazines, and newspapers were channels through which individuals contacted the national Command Trust Network, a political action group that provided information on breast implants and connected women to local support groups. In addition, some media accounts provided a link to local groups like the Tampa Bay area Silicone Sisters. Helen "heard the name Command Trust Network, I think on the *Connie Chung* show, so I contacted them." The national network also helped the women form local groups. A woman from Denver explained how it works:

It starts like this: somebody reads an article, I happened to see one of those talk shows, and they printed that Command Trust, it's an organization that's networking . . . and there's others. There's maybe 10 organizations that I'm aware of, Lupus Plastic Implant Survivor Groups and things like that. . . . but basically I saw that Command Trust thing. I sent them a 25 cent stamped envelope and they sent me back some information, and then it began to snowball.

Terry "found out about Command Trust through a magazine" but had used information gained from television news to make connections with a Tampa Bay support group: "I have other friends that are members of a support group—Silicone Sisters. . . . I saw it on the TV and I got in touch with some of the girls that . . . knew about it, and we all drove, and some people have been going to meetings for . . . couple of years." Susan found her way to the Silicone Sisters through her local paper, "It addressed . . . a group of women who were very, very ill, and how they were trying to get attention brought to this fact. . . . I decided to call the person who, who they had quoted."

Media played an important role in many women's recovery stories. Having found little help, and considerable disillusionment within the medical community, television news programs, talk shows, newspaper articles, and magazine stories emerged as crucial channels for women in diagnosing their illnesses, connecting them to support networks, providing them with health information, and guiding them to sympathetic medical care. In many cases the women believed and acted on the media reports: having implants removed, seeking contact with physicians identified in the news reports, writing to support groups named in the media accounts, contacting attorneys mentioned in the news, and writing for transcripts of the television programs.

THE ROLE OF SUPPORT GROUPS

Almost as influential as news media were the women's support networks. Terry described her local support group as a form of therapy and the national network as a source of guidance:

It's [the Silicone Sisters] like, it's like going to a psychiatrist . . . because you're sharing your experiences with other people, so I met these people through that organization, through the support group. . . . I keep in touch on the telephone with a lot of them. . . . I get newsletters from Command Trust Network which is a national group of women. . . . I found out about Command Trust through a magazine. . . . There was a big article in there and it gave the address of Command Trust and I wrote and sent them a letter and they wrote me back and, then you can get their mailings and stuff . . . what's going on with the FDA and different doctors to contact for like removal of your implants, and different people that have been through different things, new tests that are becoming available, just basically anything that has to do with any problems that anyone's had from the implants. . . . [It's a] great, great help . . . I've learned a lot. I know probably as much as maybe some of the doctors do.

Although the news media were the most important agents in the women's diagnosis stories, support networks were critical agencies for many. Terry was among half of the women we talked to who depended on local support groups for interpersonal support and/or national networks for information. Belonging to a variety of organizations including Command Trust Network, Silicone Sisters, Y-Me?, and Lupus Implant Survivors Network, the importance of the groups varied from individual to individual. For many women, the networks were critical sources of comfort and information.

The networks gave women guidance they had not found in the medical community. When Susan contacted a member of the Silicone Sisters she was directed to the FDA hearing records and to a rheumatologist specializing in silicone-related problems. Paula's support group provided names of physicians, addresses for further networking, aid in obtaining the FDA hearing records, and "different directions for help." A member of the Command Trust Network directed Jill to contact Surgitek, who subsequently paid for her implants to be removed. Donna's breast cancer support group, Y-Me?, recommended "psychiatrists who have treated other patients in the group, so that they can talk to someone personally, we have books that they can read." She concluded, "Many of the patients in the support group are learning more from the members than they are from their own doctors."

The importance of finding others suffering similar symptoms and facing comparable decisions was affirmed by many women. Susan's initial skepticism concerning the Silicone Sisters became a dramatic tale of connection and relief when she perceived that she had, after all her searching, found a source of knowledge and information. Having seen the article in the *Lakeland Ledger,* Susan called the number of a local member of the support group:

[I] decided I wasn't going to say anything to her [about my symptoms] because I didn't really want to be influenced by anything. And so I told her that I thought I, that I did have implants and I might possibly have some problems but I really wasn't familiar with anything that was going on. . . . She asked me a couple of questions, one of them, did my feet hurt? . . . and that got my attention right there. Because there was no reason for her to ask that, I mean, it's so unrelated, so totally disassociated from breasts, and . . . then I talked to her further and she mentioned that I might want to get the . . . Hearing papers and, I wrote to Washington and got, I called, and got those. And I asked her for any other help because I couldn't find anybody who would talk to me; nobody knew anything and I didn't know how to get this information. . . . She mentioned [a rheumatologist] . . . suggested I might try to call . . . I was very pleased to get at least someone knowledgeable enough to discuss this with me.

Like Susan, Jill acknowledged the importance of community shared by members of her local group. She described the mission of Y-Me?, "We really feel that it's an obligation that we have to each other to make sure that each person gets quite a bit of support."

PHYSICIANS' REACTION TO THE SILICONE DIAGNOSIS

As women were finding support from other women, most were still not receiving help from physicians. Jill found only one physician listed in the Brevard County phone book who was interested in treating her silicone-related illness, "I called everybody in the phone book . . . to see if somebody would be interested in taking me on and they said, 'No way.' . . . I called every MD in Brevard County." Jill's experience is repeated in tale after tale. Armed with a diagnosis and/or information from support groups and the media, many of the women attempted to talk with their physicians about the disease and their related problems. They told us about a variety of reactions.

Most physicians consulted by the newly diagnosed women were overtly resistent. The women told us about doctors who were unwilling to consider that silicone could be the cause of their physical problems. Karen's internist "just came out and told me that nobody feels bad [from implants], 'I've never heard it.'" When Helen asked her physician "Could it be possible that I could be reacting to the breast implant?" Her plastic surgeon said, "Absolutely not." He told her that the silicone was harmless, "Your body just gets rid of it like it would any other medication or any other body waste." Nor did she find a sympathetic ear from any other physicians she visited: "Other doctors in Minnesota are not willing to discuss that there is any connection whatsoever and that includes the University of Minnesota and the Mayo Clinic. They are vehement about it, vehement. . . ." According to Toni, that vehemence manifested itself in overt hostility toward patients:

> The medical community at large denies the existence of a connection between illness and death and silicone implants. . . . Almost all of them [are in] outright denial, kicking you out of the office, falsifying your records . . . outright denial from my plastic surgeon, completely outright denial, "Absolutely not," he said.

Some women brought news articles and support network reports with them to get their physicians' reactions. A few women told us about doctors who welcomed the additional information. Terry's physician "absolutely really knew nothing about breast implants, and I gave him a bunch of information." On a subsequent visit "he thanked me very much . . . because he was not up to date on anything that was going on [but he] was open to reading it." Having been rejected by all the other physicians in the county, Jill found a sympathetic doctor in the local Walk-In Family Clinic. She routinely takes information from the Command Trust Network to her doctor who "does whatever they say, take blood out, we send blood to Galveston, Texas, and anything it says to do, we do."

Terry's and Jill's physicians were the exceptions in the sick women's stories. Most doctors dismissed the news accounts. Donna, a nurse who previously worked for a plastic surgeon who pioneered breast implants, developed chronic pain and fatigue following her implants. Well acquainted with medical procedures, she had accumulated a significant amount of medical information and a number of news accounts related to the implant controversy. When she presented the materials to the head of rheumatology at a major medical school, the doctor rejected them because the physician "did not believe in the theory of silicone breast implants causing problems." When Donna asked the doctor about the medical research being done by physicians featured in some of the news reports, the rheumatologist said, "Those doctors do not know what they're talking about."

Other physicians were more overt in their rejection. Jill took her folder of news reports and her medial records to a physician who specialized in toxic exposure. When she and her husband explained their theory about silicone connective tissue disorder, the doctor "threw all my paperwork at me, threw it, literally." The physician said, "'You women, and you're complaining about this stuff all the time.' He goes, 'They have not proven anything.'"

After explaining the physician's reaction, Jill described his desperate, random search for any diagnosis that would discount the literature she had brought to share:

He says ... "you've got Lyme disease." And then he says, "You've been to Connecticut, haven't you?" And I said, "I've never been to Connecticut in my life." . . . He says, "Then you've been to the Carolinas." I said, "I've never been there either." You know, I'm from Ohio. And he was just, he was, he made me very angry. I thought my husband was gunna' punch him out. . . . And he had a nerve to charge me $1,020. . . . I thought I was going to faint. I mean, you know, [we had] no insurance. He knew we had no insurance, and then he runs all these . . . tests that I already had, they're in my folder. . . . He wouldn't look at them [the previous tests]. . . . [He] threw my files at me [saying], "That [silicone disease] can't be it."

Similar to Jill, Barbara searched in vain for medical help. The cumulative psychological effects of having had her unexplainable symptoms denied initially, then having her self-diagnosis of silicone disease disconfirmed, caused Barbara to be cautious when seeking subsequent medical help. She called ahead before talking to a hematologist/oncologist about her problems: "[I] asked the girl [receptionist] . . . are they [the doctors in the practice] familiar [with] and/or understand chronic fatigue syndrome, Epstein–Barr, and silicone poisoning?" She said, "Yes." Barbara asked whether the physicians were open to considerations of silicone complications, "She said they're open, they're not against them, they are open to [that diagnosis], when they ruled [out] other things." When Barbara arrived for her appointment, she was scheduled to see a new member of the practice, whose beliefs were not congruent with others in the group:

So I get the new person in the group, this Dr. X, just trained him a week ago and he doesn't believe in any of it. I asked him, do you believe in any of these things? He goes, "No, no, no, but I do believe that you're very depressed and that you need a psychiatrist."

As a result of the physician's diagnosis, Barbara discontinued her medical treatment with the oncologist, and she did not keep the appointment made for her with a psychiatrist. She explained the psychological impact of her interaction with the physician, "I got so upset that it just threw me into a real setback."

Because so many women described encounters in which doctors were resistant to information suggesting silicone was connected to a variety of complaints, we asked patients if they had any idea why physicians would react as they had. A good number of their answers pointed to profit. Several women, including Janet, told stories of conspiracy in which physicians banded together to protect their pocketbooks, "I think it's their bread and butter." Toni explained:

> There is pressure by this particular group that's making money off of implants to force the internal medicine people group with AMA pressure to not treat it, not recognize it, not send it to group studies, not deal with it, to discount it, to treat the women as if they're hysterical; "They need psychiatric treatment, they're hallucinating, they're hypochondriacs, it's not real." All of this is like, great big denial.

Helen also identified economic consideration as the motive behind the plastic surgeons' resistance to the silicone-illness link, "I think the plastic surgeons, of course, want to continue doing breast implants because it's a lucrative business." But she expanded the conspiracy to include the manufacturers: "I have heard that the Mayo Clinic is, subsidized by some company having to do with chemicals made by the companies that manufacture breast implant material." Although she admitted not knowing if the subsidies were real, she wondered how else to account for the strength of doctors' resistance to the existence of silicone connective tissue disease: "The Mayo Clinic is responding so strongly and aggressively against the idea of the implants having any connection with any kind of health problem at all, it just seems strange that they would object so strongly."

Terry's explanation broadened the conspiracy still further, including, not only the plastic surgeons and manufacturers, but other subspecialists involved in a vicious medical cycle. "The companies make money selling 'em." Following that, the "doctor makes money putting them in." When women become ill "another doctor makes the money putting them out, taking them out. Other doctors are making money trying to treat people that are sick."

SILICONE: ALIEN THREAT TO THE IMMUNE SYSTEM

Sitting by the pool at the Holiday Inn, Jean, who had traveled from Oklahoma to visit a Tampa rheumatologist, described her illness: "I've got that green slime in me. . . . It's melting . . . that's what's causing me to . . . have the pressure . . . and the choking." Despite hearing repeated denials that silicone could cause the medical complications, women like Jean developed a concrete understanding of how the silicone was affecting their bodies and why they were sick.

We were surprised and compelled by the graphic and chilling pictures of the disease which the women drew, especially given the medical consensus that silicone is an inert substance. The women's narratives portrayed silicone as an alien force that invades the body and poisons the system, "The silicone is like a foreign body, foreign matter in ya'."

In contrast to medical descriptions of silicone as inert, women portrayed silicone as a living, growing phenomenon, uncontrollable, and traveling throughout the body, "It's spreading. It's like it's taken over my heart, my lungs, my head, my whole body." Toni explained its generative properties, "that stuff (gel) bleeds slowly, it made cysts, hundreds and thousands of cysts." Barbara highlighted the penetrating properties of the gel when explaining how physicians removed the silicone which had ruptured from her implant:

> I know it's all through my system. . . . When the first time they said they had to go [searching for the gel] from here, my throat, all the way down the front of my chest to my stomach area, to my back, underneath my arm, it was, it had migrated. . . . It just kept moving . . . so they couldn't get that all out.

The moving substance was described as, not only uncontrollable, but also harmful. Karen labeled silicone a "toxin." Jill compared her body to an oil spill, overrun by poisons too enormous to be absorbed by the body:

> [Before the implant was cut] I never had any problems . . . then it just seemed to come on like a wave. . . . Maybe [before the cut] such minute amounts were seeping out that it would never have bothered me . . . your body has a built in system·and like keep it from hurting, harming other parts of your body. . . . In my case there was just too much of it thrown in all at once before my body could take over and round it all up . . . I think about it in terms of the Exxon Valdez spill you know. . . . we have oil spills in the U.S. and the environment's not hurt and the surrounding is not hurt, but for many years. . . . A minute spill can be taken care of on its own, by itself, the body will deal with it . . . clean up its own ecological parts, but gushed out, massive amounts, I don't know how.

The accounts characterized the silicone as harmful because it triggered "the immune system to act crazy." Karen called silicone an "alien disease catalyst." Toni described its actions, "It's in your system and it's stimulating your immune system to attack itself." Paula explained how her shortness of breath and recent weight loss could be the result of an immune system gone haywire, "I kinda' feel sorry for my immune system, I mean, you know, it's setting up to get rid of something that's in there, and it goes full force and yet causes problems for me, so it's trying to get rid of the silicone implants."

Despite a lack of information from physicians, some of the women we talked with were able to describe clearly how silicone acted to cause multiple symptoms. As an active toxin, the silicone was a foreign object, triggering the immune system into a futile effort to reject the implant, and finally, causing the body to turn on itself. The media appeared to have played an important role in how women came to understand their illness. Early news reports and Chung's *Face to Face* included graphic pictures of green gel-like leakage seeping from implants. These images appear in the explanations several women used to describe what was happening to the silicone in their bodies.

POSTDIAGNOSIS INTERACTIONS WITH PLASTIC SURGEONS

Based on their understanding of silicone's affect on the immune system, most of the women we talked to had decided to have their implants removed; several had already undergone the process. When women sought medical help with their removal, some experienced difficulty getting the procedures done, "None of the doctors wanna' take them out, nobody wants to help you. [They] wanna' put them in, but they don't wanna' take them out." Terry reported that after talking with several surgeons who would not remove her implants, one reluctantly agreed to perform the procedure, but subsequent attempts to schedule the procedure had failed, "He wouldn't get back with me on it, so I don't really know if he just pacified me in saying that he would take them out, but when it's coming right down to it, the man is avoiding me."

For some women, the removal process was complicated by economic problems. Most insurance companies did not recognize or pay for problems related to silicone, and surgeons were expensive. Having lost her job and collected numerous medical bills, Barbara could not afford to pay for removing and replacing her implants:

> I was just too poor to have anything done and I called everywhere. I just went crazy to know I was in so much pain and so miserable and nobody cared. . . . I mean Dr. X was a great doctor, don't get me wrong, so was Dr. Y, but they aren't going to do it for free and they weren't going to do it for what the insurance cost. They wanted more money, they wanted like twice what the insurance, so you know you kinda' get disheartened with doctors. I know that the things, I'm not stupid, I know that there's a lot of problems with . . . people suing . . . I know that, but there's gotta' be a certain amount of caring there that, I understand plastic surgeons are in the business to make money. But to be so, I guess, cold about the fact that somebody's hurting. You know, is just beyond me.

For Jean, the problem was not money. Instead, she found no plastic surgeon she could trust to replace her implants. At a local clinic, she consulted with two plastic surgeons: "They both treated me like I'd never been treated as a patient, I mean they were rude. They were abrasive [in] that their examination was extremely painful." Jean's voice dropped to a whisper when she told us, "I accused them of being queer . . . not [to] their face." She explained that "if that was a man they wouldn't be treating you [this way]." The doctors were willing to remove her implants, but indicated that they would not replace them or do follow-up surgery to deal with the aesthetic consequences. Jean reported being incredulous at their attitude. She said, "'In other words you're gonna' remove them, not put anything back in?' He said 'Yeah . . . And you'll just have a couple of empty bags hanging there.'" Having heard the prognosis, Jean thought, "Bullshit, I'm not going back to them."

When women talked about their recent interactions with plastic surgeons, some were laudatory about the surgeon's skills, others were frustrated by the physician's lack of cooperation in removing implants, but all recalled their initial contacts with plastic surgeons who failed to warn them about the medical complications of implants. As they made decisions about removing or replacing implants, the women seemed to enter a "sadder-but-wiser" mood that called forth memories of meetings in which plastic surgeons raised their hopes about the risk-free nature of the implants. The doctors failed to provide information that would have dissuaded them from having the implants. Terry "was told that mammograms would be no problem. . . . I was totally uninformed. I thought it was like Band-Aid surgery, they [the plastic surgeons] presented it like it was going to be Band-Aid surgery." Paula described her plastic surgeon as "a nice man, real good about explaining things" who told her "nothing" about risks "except that they were totally safe." Leslie explained, "You never got, the only thing you ever got told about the implants was the usual surgical complications, you know, infection, bleeding, capsulation." Nancy could not remember the plastic surgeons telling her about complications. Her husband contributed, "They certainly didn't say anything about any side effects as far as silicone was concerned."

TAKING CHARGE OF HER OWN HEALTH

> You really come to a place where it's a, it's a very trust shattering issue and it's, and it makes me angry, you really have to come to a place almost and grow up and become your own steward of your own health, and it rattles every faith you have in any of this kind of system, because you know . . . from personal experience that you cannot trust a certain segment of [doctors].

Feeling betrayed by the medical profession, Toni had taken her medical care into her own hands. She was not alone. As the women described their experience with implants, almost all came to a point when they assumed primary responsibility for their own diagnosis and decisions about their bodies. Often that decision came as a rejection of physicians as authorities and a decision to trust their own perceptions. Jean described such a turning point with one of her doctors:

> I was so sick and in so much pain I could not handle it. . . . I went back to my endocrinologist and he said, "Everything's fine." And I kept getting sick and I kept hurting more, I mean, immediately I could do weather forecasting [with swelling in my breasts]. A week before we would have a front come in, I would start having more, it's a different pain. . . . The closer a front got the worse it got . . . I literally would double over, go down to my knees . . . my headaches had gotten worse. . . . Anyway, the doctors said, "No, that's ridiculous, you can't, you can't be able to forecast weather." My mother said, "Hell, you can't." She said, "I've got arthritis, I can tell you when we've got a front coming in."

When physicians failed to affirm the women's physical experiences, their diagnoses, or their decisions, the storytellers turned to other women or their own histories, concluding that they would rather trust their personal knowledge than the doctors' expertise. Relying on friends to help her cope with debilitating symptoms, Jean declared, "I said, 'to hell with it . . . they can all go to hell; I'm not going to any more doctors.'"

Many, but not all, of the women in the study were angry with their physicians. However, all had cast aside the idealization of the physician as the final authority on their health. Even those who still maintained trust in their physicians came to a point when they took responsibility for their own health care:

> My doctors have been wonderful. . . . He says . . . "You've got to make the decision [whether to have breast implants removed], it's not mine to make. These are the studies that are done . . . this is what's new, this is what's old, you know, you've got to make the decision." They [the doctors] can't say that they do or don't believe. . . . It's not their place to say that.

Finding a cause for their illnesses, directions for help, a community of support, the women we talked to seemed empowered by the media and their support groups. Having suffered what they saw as rejection, and sometimes abuse, by the medical community, many women learned to trust other sources of information and their own experience more than the advice given to them by plastic surgeons and other physicians. Believing the implants had caused their multiple illnesses, most of these women decided, against the recommendations of the majority of physicians, to remove the devices.

IMPLICATIONS OF POSTDIAGNOSIS STORIES

Those who study the impact of communication on health have identified several functional outcomes of successful communication between doctors and patients that we find to be important in understanding the implant patients' stories and their impact on the doctor-patient relationship: the development of personal meaning for illness, a perception of support, and a feeling of control over one's body and its surroundings (Arntson, 1989; Brody, 1987; Taylor, 1983). The women's stories revealed that, in general, these needs were met outside the medical community, rather than in concert with it.

As the previous chapter demonstrates, not all diagnoses provided satisfying explanations for illness. The "illness experience must be given an explanation of the sort that will be viewed as acceptable, given the patient's existing belief system and worldview" (Brody, 1987, p. 6). Before identifying their ailments as the result of implants, many women had been told the illness was a product of their imagination or aging. These diagnoses did not fit into the women's dominant image of themselves as healthy and active. In addition, the diagnoses failed to provide a clear cause for the dramatic shift in their lives. "People are not comfortable with random events that can so profoundly affect their lives" (Arntson & Droge, 1987, p. 159).

In contrast, the diagnosis many women found in the media, relating their illnesses to silicone poisoning, provided a much more satisfying explanation. It gave a definitive time when a change occurred (rupture or leakage of the implants), imposing order on a chaotic set of events (Arntson & Droge, 1987). In addition, diagnosis of the illness as caused by silicone enabled women to identify themselves with others and to separate themselves from the ailment:

> The sociocultural dimension that plays a role in meaning . . . suggests . . . one feature of one's psychological reaction to illness is the conviction that one's illness is unique; great comfort results when the physician is able to give a name to the complaint . . . it must have an existence apart from me; so then I can struggle against it. (Brody, 1987, p. 8)

The diagnosis allows a woman to see the illness, not as a product of her thinking or lifestyle, but as a foreign invader to be combatted. The detachment of illness from one's self is clearly seen in women's descriptions of silicone as a toxic, foreign substance invading the body, causing it to fight itself. Since her problem has a name and is no longer imaginary, the patient has something concrete to resist.

Beyond explanation, patients need social support in order to create positive meaning for their illnesses. "The patient must perceive that he or she is surrounded by and may rely upon a group of caring individuals" (Brody, 1987, p. 6). Researchers in a variety of disciplines have found links between relational support and the individual's ability to handle a variety of crises, including physical illnesses, successfully (Albrecht & Adelman, 1984). Support can be manifested by giving emotional affirmation, information, assistance, and guidance.

In the women's stories, abandonment was a common theme. Doctors had not provided ongoing support; instead, women visited a variety of doctors seeking help. Some physicians had dismissed the women, sending them home with the explanation that their disease experiences were imaginary, or referring them to psychiatrists. Other physicians had avoided the women or refused to see them altogether. The physicians' failure to diagnose the symptoms as physical illnesses also contributed to the lack of social support. A diagnosis leads to caring community support only when a physician, or other health care official, offers an explanation that fits a generally accepted concept of illness (Brody, 1987). Thus, the physicians' dismissal of their symptoms as normal aging, or imagining, cost the women a network of social support. The women's stories also include gradual social isolation resulting from an inability to perform important family and community roles. Without their normal support system and finding little support from physicians, these women were missing a critical element in recovery.

Where did the women find social support? Their stories identified Command Trust Network, Y-Me?, Silicone Sisters, and other support groups. These self-help groups provided people to talk to, guidance, advice, and "therapy." An interesting dynamic occurred in the social networks, which women found helpful. During the time that some women were unable to perform as part of their normal social networks, they did find self-help groups rewarding. "The research shows that some of the most effective supporters may be those who *share a context* with the person in need" (Albrecht & Adelman, 1984, p. 7). Whereas women found themselves too depleted to connect with significant others who did not share or understand the ailments they faced, they were empowered by meeting with others who understood and shared their illnesses. "Communication with others who share the stressful context may be most effective because such individuals are more familiar with the intensity of the situation, share a common meaning for environmental symbols with the receiver, and therefore may play a special role in the uncertainty reduction process" (Albrecht & Adelman, 1984, p. 7).

Social support is closely related to the patient's need for control. Patients need a feeling of "mastery or control" over the illness (Brody, 1987, p. 6). Studies have shown a relationship between a patient's sense of control or mastery and their ability to recover from illness (Smith & Pettegrew, 1986). By providing help with actions and behaviors that enabled the patients to meet goals, the support network empowered women (Albrecht & Adelman, 1984). Local and national support groups fulfilled several important support functions for women. They modeled ways of coping with problems, provided agendas of actions women could take, removed the mystery experienced during the prediagnosis stories, and helped women to see the reason for problems and how others had dealt with them. Several women reported that the self-help groups were places where individuals could share their experiences. Such stories can serve as models showing how others dealt with problems, thus empowering the women for coping with their own difficulties (Arntson & Droge, 1987).

Sharing information, experiences, and advice all help to reduce the uncertainty involved in the disease process and help women to experience greater control over their lives and experiences. Similar functions and experiences have been found in studies of other self-help groups, including epilepsy networks (Arntson & Droge, 1987). Brody explained that patients often improve when they feel "powerful enough to affect the course of events for the better" or when they feel that some person or group aligned with them is powerful enough to effect change (Brody, 1987, p. 6). The breast implant self-help groups may function as many similar groups do, as channels of empowerment (Arntson & Droge, 1987).

In the women's stories, critical psychological needs were met, not by physicians but by the media and by self-help groups. Brody (1987) concluded that "since medicine is devoted to changing things for the better within a caring social setting, all three elements of meaning . . . [explanation, social support, and mastery] must be present for the medical encounter to be successful" (p. 8). When women did not find those needs met by their doctors, they turned to other sources.

We were struck by the powerful presence of media and support groups as influences in the women's decisions about their health care. These stories argue for the consideration of much larger contexts of medical decision making, including media, self-help groups, and other sources as influences that can override the medical advice women receive from physicians (Arntson, 1989).

Clearly, these women found information in the media and support networks more satisfying than that given to them by the majority of their doctors. The appearance of medical news in popular periodicals is likely to increase that influence. As media coverage of medical research appears with increasing frequency in popular newspapers and magazines, the public has alternate sources of information about their bodies. Complicating the process is recent media attention to the results of initial and preliminary reports, before repeated studies can confirm medical conclusions. As a result, the public is receiving increasing amounts of contradictory information about disease and treatment before the medical community has come to consensus regarding it. Research printed in the medical journals is often reported in the popular press before the professional journals hit the physician's mailbox. Patients may have read about preliminary results of studies before physicians have had time to inform themselves.

Traditionally, the physician has been a primary and respected source of health information and the gatekeeper to other specialists. As a result of increasing media coverage of health issues, patients, like the women we interviewed, may become more detached from their doctors, the traditional source of medical authority. In the case of the implant patients, the media led women to specialists, self-help groups, and other agencies that provided further information. Doctors usually perform these functions. When our interviewees took media and support group information to teach their doctors about silicone diseases, they were attempting to reverse the traditional roles. These women described themselves as knowing "as much as most doctors." These attempts challenged the typical doctor-patient relationship and its traditional power differential. Not surprisingly, some doctors resisted. If the patient is no longer dependent on the doctor for information and diagnosis, she becomes the steward of her own health. The implant recipients who felt very sick became unwilling to accept expert medical opinion that contradicted their own experiences. They accepted nonmedical opinion and assumed responsibility for their own well-being.

We found an important distinction between the doctors from whom women detached and physicians in whom women maintained their trust. Patients continued to work with physicians who admitted they were not omniscient. These physicians communicated respect for the patient's knowledge and experiences, and expressed ongoing support for the patient. Jill's story provides an example. She praised her physician even though the doctor could not find a diagnosis for the patient's illness:

> She's been following me all along. Before we knew what was wrong with me . . . she was losing her mind. She says "Gad, I've done every test I can think of and they're all coming up normal, but you're sick." She said, "I've watched you lose weight, you don't sleep at night, I can tell on days when you come in here when you haven't slept." She says, "I just don't know what's wrong." [After I heard about the problem on *Geraldo*], the Command Trust Network . . . sent me newsletters. . . . I take them immediately to my . . . doctor and she does whatever they say. . . . She said, you know "anything, if it's worth helping you let's do it."

Jill valued the attention her physician gave her and the doctor's willingness to try "anything" that might help. Rather than deny the patient's experience because the physician could not diagnose it, the doctor admitted she was stumped, but was open to learning more in order to help the patient. The physician did not make the patient feel crazy in order to make the doctor look omniscient. And the physician sent the message that she would stand by the patient through the uncertainty. The confirmation of experience and support was more important to Jill than an immediate diagnosis.

The stories told to us by women with symptoms they attributed to their silicone gel breast implants command our attention. These stories tell of loss and confusion: the loss of strength and endurance, the loss of social relationships, the loss of careers and finances, the loss of self esteem, the loss of gender, and the onset of confusion. What meaning could women give to these losses? When they turned to their doctors for interpretation and amelioration, they often found neither. The explanations offered contradicted and even denied the women's own experiences. Thus, the traditional doctor–patient relationship and the usual method of medical diagnosis and treatment failed to meet not only the women's somatic complaints, but also their psychosocial concerns and their need for meaning.

Instead of using doctors to fill their needs, many of these women turned to explanations provided by the news media and by other women in support groups. The women became stewards of their own health care. They accepted diagnoses that made sense to them, and followed treatments, including implant removal, because they believed the treatments would help. They used medical opinion only when it validated their experiences, admitted its own fallibility, and invited participation in gathering information and making choices.

We are not in a position to judge whether the women, or the physicians they rejected, are scientifically correct about the relationship between silicone and illness. We can, however, empathize with the pain and frustration the women have experienced. Clearly, they have not found solace or relief from those to whom society directs us when we hurt. Absent that help, these women, after much searching, took control of their own well being, relying on information they gleaned from the media and from other women. The lesson for medicine seems clear. The patient in distress who feels rejected will, in turn, reject the authority of those who deny the validity of her experience. She will seek other sources for meaning and help. Perhaps each of us, in much smaller ways, makes similar decisions. Listening to patients, empathizing with them, and accepting the real disruption of women's lives, may seem like platitudes to doctors. But the stories we heard could not have occurred if these patients felt those platitudes had been given life.

Of course, not all women with implants are like those we studied in the last two chapters. Not all, not even most, believe their implants have made them ill. Statistically, the vast majority of women with implants are happy, not distressed, with them. Their stories are presented in the next chapter along with the differences in the way satisfied women relate what has happened in their lives.

4

STORIES OF SUCCESS
AND SATISFACTION

The stories of the women we talked to who blame illness on their implants compel our interest and our compassion. These women have suffered, both from their symptoms, and from their inability to find meaning on which to build understanding and acceptance of their experiences. However, these women are not the norm among those with breast implants. By all accounts, the vast majority of implant patients not only fail to see themselves as ill, but are pleased with their implants. Surely an understanding of the communication surrounding silicone gel breast implants must take their experiences into account.

To obtain that perspective, we interviewed 15 women who described themselves as satisfied with their implants between 1992 and 1994. Obtaining interviews with these women was more difficult than with those who linked illnesses to their implants. Women who were satisfied with their implants were not likely to be in contact with their plastic surgeons or rheumatologists. Nor were they visible in support groups such as the Silicone Sisters. As a result, our interview roster developed slowly through word of mouth. Consequently, many of the women we interviewed were friends, linked by more commonalities than their implant experiences. We interviewed five women who lived in the same high-rise condominium. Three of the women we talked to were doctors' wives and two others worked in the medical field. It was not unusual in our interviews to hear references to the lives and stories of other women we had interviewed previously. During one session, the interviewee told us that a woman we had interviewed months before had been diagnosed with breast cancer. We felt, in a way, as though we had become a part of a network and a community. Most women in this group were well educated and affluent.

In other ways, like the women described in the previous two chapters, the satisfied women were diverse; their ages ranged from late 20s to mid-60s. Frances[1] had her first set of implants in 1972. Elizabeth had her first set of expanders in place at the time of the interview. We interviewed several women by telephone, allowing us to expand the study geographically beyond Tampa. One of our interviewees was a cocktail waitress in Las Vegas, another was a nurse in Jacksonville, Florida.

---

[1]As in the previous chapters, we have changed the women's names to protect their confidentiality

Especially important is the diversity in types of implants chosen by these satisfied women. Five had pure silicone implants; one woman had a double lumen implant that was primarily silicone; two women had double lumen implants that were about 70% saline; seven women had saline-filled implants in silicone envelopes.

The collective stories of the satisfied women represented in this chapter reflect a difference in women's foci and priorities as they reconstructed their experiences. Our use of open-ended questions encouraged women to concentrate their attention and time on what was important to them. Sick women emphasized the pain of illness related to their implants and their search to overcome it. Their before–after stories were narratives of once active lives now diminished. The satisfied women also told before–after stories, but they explained them in problem-solution formats, where the implants were part of the solution for four different problems: fibrocystic disease, family histories of breast cancer, cancer-related mastectomies, and small breasts. Plastic surgeons were agents of the desired change.

MOTIVATIONS FOR IMPLANTS

The "before" stories center on the women's reasons for having implant surgery. Motivations were the same for women who are satisfied and women who are sick, but the two groups' stories differ in emphasis and detail. Differences are found, not in why the two groups chose to have implants, but in the amount of time they spent talking about motivation rather than illness. For satisfied women, the reasons were significant; they played a central role in the implant story. For the sick women, motives for having implants were secondary to the illness experience and to the healing process. Satisfied women highlighted their reasons for having implants. This section on motivation, although told in the stories of the satisfied women we interviewed, is also representative of the more abbreviated motivation stories of the women who are ill. Although their motivations were similar, the stories of the satisfied women became markedly different from those of sick women following the section on motivation. It is important to note that the differences in the collective stories represented here might not be due to variations in what happened, but rather, in what each group thought important enough to relate.

Breast Augmentation

Most breast implant surgery is performed to enhance the size of women's breasts rather than to replace breasts removed by mastectomy. Estimates vary from 67% to 80%. Similarly, breast enlargement was the most common motive for the women we interviewed. Fifteen of the 35 women we spoke to had breast augmentation. They had implants to compensate for perceived inadequacies in what nature had provided them, to correct asymmetrical or misshapen breasts, and/or to regain the size and shape that pregnancy and nursing had diminished. Unlike the images promoted by fashion magazines and tabloids, the majority of these women were not hoping for Dolly Parton sized breasts, but to erase the emotional damage of being flat chested in a world that favored well-endowed women. Marie's story is typical of the women who had implants for augmentation purposes. She described herself as "flatchested." "I had always been *extremely* insecure about that." Although Marie began to develop breasts early, she traced her insecurity about breast size to an early episode with her first bra:

> [My mother] got my first bra for me when I began to develop, you know, it was like I started to develop and then I stopped. . . . I budded early but then nothing else. And she got my first bra for me. Well, I couldn't quite fill it out. . . . Well, what *she* did, coming from the era that she came from, she got a pair of her falsies. She wasn't particularly a large-breasted woman. And she cut them down, you know, shaped them up, and said, "Well, just put them in there." Well, I did and it was great. You know, I was 11 years old and just great. But you can't wear them one day and then none the next, you know. And it's sort of like you know, when you dye your hair, you know. . . . You can't not do it once in awhile. You know, you just have to keep it up. Well, I didn't know that. And, you know I went to school one day and I felt just great and really grown up. And then the next day and the next day. And then, after about a week, I thought, "This is getting old." You know. And they were hot. And I thought, "God, I can't appear flatchested now." So, it just stuck. And there it was.

Marie's early "deception" led to acute self-consciousness about her breast size at home and at school. Afraid her family would find out she was not developing normally, she even slept in her bra. Describing the potential horrors of the school shower room, Marie exploded, "Oh, no way! You know, I'd just stick my leg in there, stick my arm in there, throw a little water under my arms. But no way!"

Her attempts to appear normally endowed did not always succeed, causing excruciatingly painful moments for Marie as an anxious teen:

> One of my terrible memories from my teenage years was, you know, the old-fashioned bathing suits·I had falsies in there and, of course, you go in the water and they absorb the water and the rest of your suit dries in a while but the falsies don't. And a guy hugged me. And he had on a freshly starched shirt, you know, and he was leaving and when he hugged me this water squished out and left these two wet spots on his shirt. I was mortified. I think I was about 14. And, I must say, though, that it kept me from being promiscuous. You know, there was *no way* that I was going to do that. And, so, you know, I guess it has it's advantages.

Like Marie, many of the women who had breast augmentation felt stigmatized at an early age and had suffered (real or imagined) teasing from peers and their families. Common in many of their stories were apprehensions about revealing clothing, especially swimsuits, which brought the anxieties to a head. Marie revealed that even after she was married, "I wasn't comfortable in a bathing suit."

The difficulties of finding a suitable swimsuit appeared in almost all the augmentation interviews. Leanne described the problem as a primary reason for getting her implants. When she decided to move to Florida, she realized she would be spending "half my life in a swimsuit." Ashley described her preimplant appearance in skimpy "summer-type clothing" as "just atrocious." With one breast noticeably smaller than the other, "I would find that I was very self-conscious about it, especially in a swimsuit, and to the point where I could hardly get a swimsuit top to fit me."

Another common problem expressed by augmentation patients was feeling out of proportion. Besides being flatchested, Marie described herself as "tall for my age at the time, and . . . I felt big. But then here's this flat chest. And it really just didn't seem to go together." Leanne explained that her breasts were out of proportion with the rest of her body: "I grew up as a fairly flat chested girl and everything else, proportionately, everything else was in very nice shape. I mean, I'm blonde-haired, blue-eyed, and had a nice figure . . . [I felt] inadequate. I felt like I was missing something." As a result of her implant surgery, she reported feeling as if her body was correctly proportioned for the first time. "I feel like for my body weight, and my posture, and my build, and my muscle makeup, that I just feel normal."

Augmented women often recalled feeling sexually and romantically inhibited before their implants. After Marie explained that her implants had prevented her from being promiscuous as a teenager, she wistfully continued that even after her marriage, "I didn't feel like a woman . . . I didn't feel feminine. . . . It became an issue for me sexually. I just didn't feel, you know, very sexual or sensual in that regard." Ashley echoed this same concern, previous to the implants "any kind of intimate relationship that I had . . . I certainly was very, I don't know what word to use, very nervous and self-conscious about it."

Feelings of inadequacy and inhibition were usually internal, "personal." Some women described social harassment as well. Tonya recalled jogging with a friend when she was 25. "Cruisers" passing by in a car yelled to her out the window, "Are you a girl or a guy?" The recollected pain was clear in her voice as she remembered when she used to pull on a T-shirt and the only protrusions were her nipples. Amy's embarrassment began at home in her teens when her father made comments about her flat chest. The criticisms continued for years. When she went to work as a cocktail waitress in Las Vegas, her boss commented, "You are as cute as shit, if you only had boobs." She had implants shortly after that.

The embarrassment of being flat chested was the motivation for Marie, Leanne, Elaine, Julia, Amy, Ashley, and Tonya to have breast implants. It compelled many women whose stories were told in the last two chapters as well: Jill, Donna, Carol, and Terry. Janine, Barbara, and Toni had implants after pregnancy and nursing had diminished their once full figures. Helen had implants to make her breasts more symmetrical and surgery to remove too many nipples.

Breast Cancer Reconstruction

The second most common reason for implants was to reconstruct breasts lost to cancer surgery. Ten women, two who were satisfied with their implants and eight who blamed their illness on them, had chosen reconstruction following mastectomies. The desire to appear normal, following radical surgery common in these stories, was presented by Irene:

> Mine was not really for how I looked, you know, it's not really something, like, cosmetic. It's more because I had cancer. And I had decided before I had even surgery for the malignancy, that I wanted this done, that I did not want to wear those [prostheses]. . . . I found out on . . . Tuesday that I had cancer and I had the surgery Thursday. And on Wednesday I had an appointment with the plastic surgeon and went in, and he showed me various pictures of what he had done to other patients. . . . I felt very strongly that I wanted my life to get back to as normal as it was and that I wanted some sort of bosoms; I didn't want very much because I didn't have very much to begin with. So I really wanted to sort of, to look like I did before I started this. . . . I had a double mastectomy. But when you have that you're concave, you're not just flat . . . You are indented.

The desire to return to normalcy is a strong part of the reconstruction patient's story. The appearance of the mastectomy scar is for some women an unpleasant reminder of disease. Even Patricia, whose mastectomy scar "didn't bother" her, remarked, "I felt it was an ugly sight . . . not a normal sight."

Of the group of women who were satisfied with their implants, only Irene and Patricia had breast cancer reconstruction. Eight women who complained about implant-related health problems were cancer reconstruction patients: Melanie, Leslie, Karen, Mary, Nancy, Paula, Jean, and Harriet.

Prophylactic Mastectomies

Closely related to the reconstruction stories are the accounts of women who underwent preventive mastectomies, because they were fearful of family histories filled with breast cancer or were tired of multiple biopsies caused by fibrocystic disease. Although controversial, subcutaneous mastectomies were performed by plastic surgeons who removed most of the breast tissue as a means of reducing a woman's chances of having breast cancer or to eliminate chronic biopsies and aspirations caused by fibrocystic disease. Nine women had undergone prophylactic mastectomies and subsequent implantation surgery. Rachel, Elizabeth, Lorraine, Gillian, and Frances were satisfied with their implants. Ann, Janet, Susan, and Sarah are among the women whose stories were told in previous chapters and believed the procedures they had to save their lives now threatened them.

Preventive Mastectomies to Avoid Breast Cancer.   One of the most powerful elements of these women's stories is the fear of breast cancer. The emotion permeates some of the women's sense of identity. Rachel began her interview stating, "I am a high cancer risk." She traced breast cancer through her female relatives, ending the interview by drawing a grim picture of her legacy:

> My grandmother died of cancer of the breast at age 50 when she shouldn't have and nobody knew anything about it. They cut her breasts off on the kitchen table with a kitchen knife and my father heard her screaming, running away from the house. They gave her a shot of whiskey.

Now in her 50s, Rachel had undergone preventive double mastectomies, beyond subcutaneous procedures, removing the nipples and areolas as well as the breast tissue to prevent "a horrible death." She concluded firmly, "If you don't have breast tissue, you don't die of cancer of the breast."

Although 20 years younger than Rachel, Elizabeth had similar experiences watching her sister, mother, and aunt die terrible cancer deaths:

> I have a strong history of breast cancer in my family. My sister just passed away in March. My mother passed away in '85 and I've had two aunts that have also had it. One died very young, at 33, and the other one just had her second mastectomy last year. So it's real strong. There's no other women in my family.

Elizabeth had been very close to her sister throughout her illness; driving her to the doctor, intervening with indifferent physicians, and watching her growing disability. Elizabeth described the physical toll the illness had taken:

> Her lips were cracking; her mouth got sores all in it. Eating certain foods and she'd just, you know, lose it an hour later or something like that. . . . She started to have to wear a wig . . . had all this gel and stuff all over [her mouth] . . . It was hard to talk. . . . She got really self-conscious.

In her last days, Elizabeth's sister was in too much pain to drive herself to see her physician. Elizabeth and her husband drove her there, and Elizabeth recounted her sister's terrible cough and awful pain as she cried and screamed in the car.

With her sister's death only a few months past, Elizabeth predicted her own situation unless she had a mastectomy: "I was told by my radiologist that I have a 50 to 70% chance of getting it since every woman had it before menopause." Having watched her female family members die of cancer, despite the reassurances of oncologists and the newest cancer research, Elizabeth was skeptical of the medical community's ability to help people like herself: "So I decided to have them removed and get implants put in because I didn't trust oncologists who, in the past, have always said, 'We think we got it all.' And yet it comes back again a year or two later and there's nothing you can do."

Elizabeth described how, following mastectomies, her mother's breast cancer reoccurred in her spine. Her sister's "traveled to her lymph nodes on the same side as her mastectomy." One aunt's cancer reoccurred in the other breast. A second aunt's cancer spread to her lungs. In each case, "all the conventional things would only delay it . . . This is no cure. . . . Why should I risk it and just pretend and have all this hope and trust these people when I've firsthand experience it does not work?"

During the 2 years of her sister's illness, Elizabeth began to gather information about breast cancer and its treatments. She insisted, despite medical convention, on having a mammogram during her 20s. She talked with her sister-in-law who had prophylactic mastectomies and implants 10 years previously to rid herself of fibrocystic disease. Her sister-in-law told her, "They're great. I don't even think about them anymore." After consulting with multiple physicians, she finally found a radiologist who convinced her that the American Cancer Society was not making much progress with younger women who have breast cancer. "If you take the women under 40 who get it, no, we're not making any progress in that." His opinion confirmed Elizabeth's own assessment, "Obviously, my family could testify to that."

Elizabeth had already entertained the idea of having a preventive mastectomy. The radiologist recommended that she investigate the possibility further. After consulting with a surgeon who also thought the procedure was a good idea, she claimed, "It just kind of snowballed from there. I saw the plastic surgeon and she started talking about what she could do for me and everything else. I went from there."

As she went through the process, Elizabeth's sister-in-law and other women who had undergone this same procedure confirmed her decision and told her what to expect:

> She pretty much told me what to expect as far as the procedure goes and how she felt at some different points. . . . I think if you talk to somebody who's already experienced it and ask them what changes have you gone through, what's really different after everything . . . you know what to expect. That helped a lot.

Preventive Mastectomies for Women With Fibrocystic Disease.

Like Elizabeth's sister-in-law, Lorraine, Sarah, Susan, and Frances had mastectomies to remove fibrocystic disease with its painful lumps and chronic biopsies. Frances began having trouble with cysts in her breasts in 1964. Unable to distinguish malignancies from benign lumps, she underwent repeated biopsies, which at that time required 3-day hospital stays. "Very concerned" that the lumps might be cancer, Frances felt she could not ignore them. After 8 years and many surgeries, her physician suggested an experimental treatment being performed at Walter Reed Hospital, removing breast tissue and replacing it with implants. "Tired of having so many biopsies," Frances was glad to be a part of the experiment.

In 1985, Lorraine found herself in a similar situation, "I had so many cysts that [the surgeon] couldn't tell the cysts from the breast tissue." She had needle biopsies every 2 weeks, "They stick that needle in you five times and aspirate you . . . you get to the point where you can't take much more of that either." During one biopsy, the surgeon found tissue "in the stages that he'd seen several, many times before it went into a malignancy." After Lorraine had endured 8 years of worry and pain, her surgeon advised her to have a prophylactic mastectomy. Lorraine's sister had also suffered from fibrocystic disease and had previously undergone mastectomies and implants. After talking with her sister, her husband, and a number of physicians, Lorraine decided, "It was better than facing a malignancy later on down the road, so I went ahead and had it done."

A crucial part of Lorraine's decision was the availability of implants following the mastectomy:

Prior to having it done, I went to a plastic surgeon . . . and I talked with him about the implants because I definitely wanted them . . . for my own sanity. . . . I knew from the time, after I had the mastectomy, that, that I would never probably be happy with myself unless I had the implants done. And I think it's sort of a self-esteem thing for a woman, you know, it makes you feel like a whole person.

She described her sense of loss during the period while she was waiting for the implants:

You just didn't feel like you're all there, you know, you just, it, my clothes didn't . . . fit. It was just that, you know, I looked so sunked in, you know you could tell that I didn't have anything, and it was sort of surprising. . . . I came home from the hospital and my husband said, "Let me see what you look like," and I said "No." I said, "I cannot believe what, what I look like, what a person looks like, what a woman looks like without breast tissue. And I just could not wait till the day came that I could have something done."

Frances echoed Lorraine's feelings about the implants. Although she is a petite woman and she "never had much there" as breasts, Frances said she did not know if she would have had the preventive mastectomy if implants had not been available. Their value to her is evident by the fact that she has had her implants replaced twice due to hardening over the past 20 years.

Whether the women had their implants for enhancement, breast cancer reconstruction, or prevention, some repeated themes characterize the women's common concerns and experiences. The patients wanted to appear as normal females. For most of them, normal women had breasts—not large—but something. Flat chested, Elaine revealed that she had waited for years "to look a little bit more normal. . . . I was always self-conscious." After her mastectomy, Rachel explained that she didn't feel like a mature woman, more like "a little girl." She explained the loss, "Breasts are important to a woman to feel feminine and total. . . . There's just a few things [including breasts] that make us feel totally feminine." Her conclusion is echoed through almost all our interviews. The reflection is reminiscent of the sick women who have had their implants removed and concluded that they have lost their gender.

Prostheses and padded bras were overwhelmingly rejected by women as a means for attaining or recovering a sense of normal femininity. When her implants leaked after 17 years, Marie spent a few weeks wearing padded bras while waiting for her new implant surgery:

> The three weeks from the time I had the "blowout" to the time that I had the surgery, I really hated that because I was having to use . . . I would use a shoulder pad, you know, in my bra to fill it out. I'd have to be very careful what I wore. And so, and I thought, it reminded me of the olden days when I used to have to go around with the padded bras and the padded bathing suits and things. And I thought, "I don't want any part of that any more."

Prostheses appeared to be no more welcome among the mastectomy patients than padded bras and falsies were to augmentation patients. Irene explained that even with a prosthesis, you don't look normal, "Even when you wear those prostheses, it's just, it's weird, it's just a different look, and I didn't want that." Gillian came to the same conclusion, for a different reason:

> I don't want to be bothered with it [a prosthesis]. I don't want it slipping and I don't want to have to worry about putting them in and out. I don't want to put on a bathing suit and have to worry about where they are. No, I don't want to be bothered. It's too much bother.

Elizabeth and Rachel did not wear prostheses themselves but their relatives and friends with similar mastectomies convinced them that prostheses were not desirable. Rachel was most concerned about the weight of the devices:

> I have friends that can't wait to get back home at five o'clock to take out their prostheses. . . . Even those with, with one prosthesis . . . Now it's deforming to their shoulder because the bra digs into it the way that women with very heavy breasts have to suffer [with the shoulder.]

Elizabeth's aunt gave her niece the same impression, "My aunt . . . hates them. . . . They're so heavy and . . . they give her rashes because they're so hot. And she hates wearing them. As soon as she gets home, it's throw on a sweatshirt type of thing."

Beyond weight and appearance, Rachel explained the prostheses would be impossible to keep in place with a double mastectomy, "You can't . . . hold down a bra with prostheses in it. . . . There's nothing to hold it down. . . . You have to have straps to attach it to panties or girdles or waistbands."

Also common to these stories is a desire to have normal-sized breasts. Like Irene, most of the women who had reconstructive surgery just wanted the size they had before surgery, "I wanted my life to get back to as normal as it was, and . . . I wanted some sort of bosoms; I didn't want very much because I didn't have very much to begin with." Even women who had augmentation surgery did not choose large implants. Amy went from an AA cup to an A cup to fit her slender frame; she wears a size 1 dress. When pressured by others to go larger, several women resisted. Patricia went from a 32A to a 34B. Her fiance' encouraged her to choose a larger implant, "36 or 38 or something! Good gracious. . . . That would have been ridiculous." When Tonya's plastic surgeon suggested that she could accommodate larger implants than the ones she requested, Tonya asked for "the smallest implant I can get, just enough to fill out my bathing suit top." Tonya explained that she just wanted to look "normal," to "fit in." Having been harassed and the focus of attention because she was too small, Tonya did not want to be the focus of attention following her implants, "I wouldn't want to be . . . somebody that all the guys looked at."

Whether the women had implants for augmentation to increase self-esteem, as reconstruction following mastectomies, as part of preventative measures against breast cancer, or to erase the worries of family cancer histories, all of our interviewees saw the implants as important solutions to urgent problems. The women were motivated by feelings of inadequacy, social embarrassment, fear, worry, and abnormality. For others, the feelings were physical, the pain of unending biopsies. They chose implants to erase those feelings and anxieties.

THE DECISION PROCESS

Having described their reason for choosing implants, the women's stories focused on other parts of the decision process. Five themes emerged in this stage of the stories: (a) For most women, the decision came at the end of lengthy deliberation. For none, was the decision to have implants a sudden whim or impulse. (b) During the period of making the decision regarding implants, interviewees spoke to other women who had implants to get advice. (c) Although the decision to have the implants was lengthy, the selection process for a plastic surgeon was more expedient. Women relied on physicians with whom they had long-term connections and with whom the women felt personally comfortable. (d) Trust in their plastic surgeons appeared to result from the initial contact when the physicians spent time with the patients answering questions, explaining alternatives, and describing procedures. (e) During the decision process, many women rejected some of the medical advice given to them and asserted their own control and choice over their health care.

The Long Wait

Most of the women we talked to thought about the possibility of having implants for a long time before having the procedure. Rachel began collecting information about breast cancer and prevention 10 years before she had her prophylactic mastectomy. Her husband, a dermatologist, clipped medical journal articles about cancer, implants, and safety: "We did quite a bit of research . . . I think I contacted about 16 different physicians then made the decision to go ahead and particularly after my sister had breast cancer and then she had some reconstruction . . . and have been 100% pleased."

By the time she made the decision to have the implants, Rachel had "a pretty thick file on things that were coming out in the medical journals."

Although her process was not as involved as Rachel's, when Elaine decided to have augmentation she also considered it for several years before she acted:

> I had thought about it for a long time and finally it was the time to do it. . . . It was not a spur of the moment idea. I've been to a consult probably a couple of years prior. I went to the surgeon who actually did it. And then I thought about it for a couple more years and thought, well, it was time.

Elaine's story is typical of the augmentation patients. Ashley, Leanne, Amy, Julia, and Marie thought about the procedure for years before they had the implants. For many, money played a major role in the delays. Wanting implants since college, Leanne waited until she had a large enough salary as an attorney to pay for the procedure. Amy received compensation from an accident, and Tonya received a small inheritance on the death of a relative. Each used the money to buy normal-sized breasts after years of feeling inadequate.

The Influence of Other Women Who Had Implants

During the period of consideration, our interviewees sought the opinions and experiences of women they knew who had implants. Just as Elizabeth's sister-in-law's and Rachel's sister's good experiences influenced their decisions to have implants, almost every woman we talked to had consulted someone she knew who had implants before she had the procedure herself. For Marie, a friend's example was a turning point:

> It was after I married . . . a good friend of mine that I'd grown up with called me up one day and said, "Guess what I did?" or "Guess what I'm going to do?" And she was a big girl. She's larger, taller than myself. And so I said, "Well, let me know how you do. . . . Let me see the results." So when she came over and showed me the results, I was so impressed. I was so impressed. And my husband said, "Would you like to do that?" And I said, "I think I would. I think I would." And she described the procedure to me and the recuperation. And I thought about it and then I made an appointment with the doctor.

Julia and Amy both had sisters whose implants had been successful. Julia said she told her plastic surgeon "I wanted my sister's [implants]. I felt like my sister's implants . . . were probably the prettiest I had ever seen." When Julia talked with other women, they reported being "perfectly satisfied." Leanne received positive confirmation about implants from an acquaintance's sister, "I didn't actually speak to her, but she said that her sister was very happy and had it done." Amy remembered her mother's implants as "awesome." The women who influenced our interviewees during their deliberations had uniformly positive experiences with their implants.

Choosing a Plastic Surgeon

Once women decided to have implants, the choice of a plastic surgeon was swift. Many of the women consulted only one surgeon. Although several women described the strong professional credentials of the surgeons they chose, other factors were more prominent in their stories. For several, the decision was made on the basis of long-term association with the doctor or the institution she or he represented. Marie, Patricia, and Lorraine chose physicians who had performed medical procedures for them in the past and were pleased with their work. However, the relationships described in several cases were more than professional. Lorraine, Janine, and Gillian described their associations with their plastic surgeons as trusted family friendships.

Lorraine's explanation emphasized the commonality in heritage and enduring contact with her physician:

> We go a long way back. He's originally from North Carolina, we are too, and we even went to school at the University of North Carolina. . . . We started going to him and I can't even remember, I guess the first time I went to him was, you know, with this, with the problem of the fibrocystic disease, because I found the lump and I went to a gynecologist and he referred me to Dr. X and I, you know, like I said, I saw him for 8 years before I had this done. . . . My husband went to him for some minor things too and we just got to know him . . . because he was just like a good ole' home town doctor, you know.

In Janine's case, she and her husband had been personal friends with the plastic surgeon and his family long before she went to him for medical assistance:

> I have known [the plastic surgeon and his wife] for years. . . . We all used to live over in [the same neighborhood] and I happened to call his wife and I talked to her about it because she had mentioned that [the physician] had told her that's what she ought to do. . . . My faith in him was impeccable and I've known him for 20 years. . . . We have children that are friends.

In Gillian's case, her loyalty was directed not toward an individual doctor, but toward the medical institution where she returned for medical care, including reconstructive surgery:

> I relied on Duke University. I did not go beyond Duke University. . . . We are Duke people, I guess is probably why. And knowing that my father-in-law had cancer of the prostate. . . . This was years ago and it was in the formative stages the cancer of giving the male hormone, removing the testicle, and they kept him alive for 11 years because he had surgery here and it reoccurred and went up there and he was alive for 11 more years and we just have a lot of confidence. It's our school and we do have a lot of confidence in it.

The sense of identification and long-term relationship embedded in these descriptions reflect feelings of trust and comfort. Although not all of the women had enduring associations with the plastic surgeons that Janine, Gillian, Marie, Lorraine, and Patricia had, many described positive rapport in their shorter relationships with their plastic surgeons.

Several women commented about how comfortable they felt with their physicians. Frances described her plastic surgeons as "compassionate and kind." When Leanne received a referral from the University of South Florida College of Medicine, she "went in for a consultation and I liked him right away. I felt real comfortable with him. . . . He was just helpful and he was friendly. . . . He was very honest to me . . . . He was very sensitive to my concerns." Amy reported feeling "very comfortable" with her surgeon from the onset. Elizabeth described her doctor as "just a nice guy . . . I felt at ease."

Descriptions of the plastic surgeon's interactions with their patients provide an explanation for why the women felt so comfortable. Plastic surgeons were consistently described as good sources of information; they answered questions, were thorough in their explanations, and communicated their ongoing concern and availability to their patients.

Women consistently praised their plastic surgeons for answering all their questions, contrary to the experiences of the sick women. Elizabeth explained the difference between her good experience with her plastic surgeon and the poor relationship her sister had with a physician, "Any questions I had, [my surgeon] answered them for me. So I felt at ease and I think that was a big difference·feeling at ease before you go in and having all your questions answered." Irene said her physician answered her questions and provided her with written materials: "He answered any question that I wanted answered and there was certainly lots of literature there for me to read." Elaine made her decision about her surgeon after only one consultation, "He was just very helpful about questions I might have."

Beyond answering questions, plastic surgeons were described as taking the time to thoroughly explain and explore options with their patients. Patricia did not remember what information she received, but she did recall the thoroughness of the explanations, "I don't remember what he told me, but he was very thorough before I went into this." Frances described the plastic surgeons and other physicians at Walter Reed Hospital who talked to her for a long time about the prophylactic procedure, explaining its experimental nature and how it was done.

The women also recalled discussions when plastic surgeons explored the benefits and limitations of different kinds of implants. They were impressed with the time the doctors took to accomplish that goal. Janine's physician even had her hold different implants:

> We asked about the advantages and disadvantages of each one. And he was very, very helpful. My gosh, we took, we must have been in there an hour and a half. Well, that's a long time, you know going over each one. . . . I couldn't tell the difference in the two implants. He gave me one of each and I couldn't tell the difference. . . . He brought them in and laid them out on the table and everything. We went over size and texture, the benefits, the disadvantages, and the health risks. He was very, very helpful.

Sometimes the doctor included unpleasant news in their thorough explanations, but patients expressed appreciation for the forewarnings. When Elizabeth asked, "What am I going to experience and how am I going to look?" The surgeon showed her pictures and reference books: "And she was honest. I mean, she said, you know, 'It's going to be painful. It's going to take about 3 to 4 months for the whole thing to be over with.' But I'm glad I knew that rather than her telling me something else."

Elizabeth was impressed that her plastic surgeon explained the difficulties as well as the benefits of the operation. Other women described physicians whose consultations included warnings that breast augmentation was not appropriate for all reasons or for all women. Ashley recounted her experience:

He asked me . . . why did I want to do it? . . . I think he wanted to make sure that I didn't think it was going to change my life dramatically. Like it would just make me this you know, Miss America kind of person. . . . He went into showing me all kind of photos before and after and, of course, explained all the risks and all that kind of thing . . . And just wanted me to make sure I had time to think about it, so I kind of went in for a consultation before I actually set up the surgery date and then there was still a pretty good period in there so that if I did have any change of mind, it wouldn't be a problem to back out. So it wasn't like he was forceful or anything like that, oh that was nice.

Like Ashley's doctor, Marie's plastic surgeon inquired about her reasons for the surgery. His questions rested primarily on her relationship at home:

He said, "Are you doing this for your husband?" and I said, "No!" . . . I said, "Not at all. This is for me. I have the full support of my husband." He said, "Are you getting ready to get a divorce?" And I said, "I have no intentions of it." And he said, "Well, a lot of women come in here and they want to have it done just before their divorce. And their husband pays for it and they're out there with a new body." He was real concerned about that.

The plastic surgeons described in the satisfied women's stories took time with patients; answering their questions, thoroughly explaining procedures and options, and sometimes even exploring motivations. Many women reported that the doctors also communicated ongoing availability and concern.

Rather than perceiving the plastic surgeon's concern as a short-term effort, the women's stories included interactions in which the physician demonstrated his or her intentions to "be there" for the patient in case of further questions or concerns. Lorraine saw her plastic surgeon many times before the surgery. She described him in those multiple interactions as "very thorough." When Leanne had complications with her implants, her plastic surgeon took the initiative to call the manufacturers and investigate possible links. Elaine's plastic surgeon gave her a number she could call if she had any questions, and later treated her for unrelated problems.

The positive doctor–patient experiences that many women described provide a compelling explanation for the fact that 9 of the 15 women did not seek a second opinion from any other plastic surgeon. For Janine, Elaine, Patricia, Gillian, Amy, Marie, Ashley, Tonya, and Elizabeth, their plastic surgeons had earned their trust.

Asserting Control Over Medical Decisions

Although the majority of women who were satisfied with their implants expressed trust in their plastic surgeons and other physicians, they did not follow all medical advice and sometimes directly disagreed with their physicians, asserting their control over their medical decisions. Unlike many women who were sick and took charge of their health care late in the implant stories, the satisfied women told us about confrontations with their physicians that happened early in the decision-making process.

Lorraine clearly expressed the opinion of most satisfied women, "I think a woman has the right to make a choice of how she wants to, what she wants to do with her body." Elizabeth enacted Lorraine's philosophy when choosing her type of implants, resisting her surgeon's preferences:

> Actually, my plastic surgeon wanted me to go with silicone because she said she likes the appearance better and she says they feel more like something that's natural. And she must have asked me three times, even though I kept saying, "No, I don't want them. No, I don't want them." She kept asking me. And she said, "Okay. I'll order the other kind." So, she just likes the appearance. . . . That's her business·making you look as best as you can. She wasn't really into the medical aspect about it but she was curious and wanted to make definitely sure that I didn't want them.

Both Elizabeth and Rachel met considerable resistance in their decisions to have preventive mastectomies; several doctors attempted to talk them out of the procedure. In each case, the women steadfastly pursued their goal in spite of the advice they received from the physicians they respected. When Elaine asked a physician for a referral to a plastic surgeon for augmentation, the doctor tried to discourage her from the procedure. She persisted in the face of his disagreement until she got a referral. In Irene's case, she got her plastic surgeon to move up the date on her implant surgery, despite his advice that she should wait.

In many stories, women who generally trusted and respected their doctors maintained control over decisions about what procedures they would have and when they would occur. Rachel articulated the spirit of these actions, "I am in control of what happens to my own body. I can turn down any suggestion by any doctor. I never have to take an IV. I never have to take any kind of medicine; there's nothing that I *have* to do."

AFTER THE IMPLANT SURGERY

The vast majority of comments we heard about the effects of implant surgery were positive. Lorraine explained that her implants have been "wonderful." Julia said that she "thoroughly enjoyed having the implants." Elaine said, "It was great." The degree to which the implants changed women's lives varied, but all of the women pointed to specific areas in their lives when the implants made a positive difference. In Leanne's case, the differences were dramatic and pervasive:

> [The implants are] terrific. I mean, I couldn't have done better myself if I had been able to draw a picture and do it myself. I enjoy the beach. I enjoy shopping. I fit into everything proportionately. I look nice. And my clothes—it's just a big difference. I mean. I feel more confident. . . . Big, big difference. I'm real happy, I mean, I wouldn't change it for anything.

Not all the women expressed such broad changes brought about by the implants. However, many told us about their increased self-esteem, the increased comfort they felt in their clothing, and a new freedom in how they dressed.

Increased Self-Esteem

For women who felt inadequate and others traumatized by surgery, implants provided a boost in self-confidence, "I feel my self-confidence level is extremely better. You know so it's definitely made a positive [difference] as far as my self-image goes." Julia reported feeling "better about myself . . . not as self-conscious." For Amy, her self-esteem increased because she "felt a little more like [a] female" and she was harassed less. The change in Tonya's self-confidence was more dramatic, "[The implants] changed my whole way of thinking about myself. . . . My life was just like, miserable, before the implants."

Irene explained how her self-esteem was connected to a restored sense of wholeness following her mastectomy:

> So I just really wanted to, sort of, to look like I did before I started this, and I'm very happy with the result. . . . And I just think it's, it's sort of a self-esteem . . . thing for a woman, you know, it makes you feel like a whole person. I don't even think about them now. . . . Nobody knows [about my surgery] unless I tell them that I have had it.

Clothing

Fit.   Women spoke a good deal about the changes that implants made in how their clothes fit. They reported that they were less self-conscious about what they wore and were more comfortable in their clothes. For some women, the fit of their clothes was a primary reason for having implants. That was the case for Rachel, who reported that the implants helped her to "feel very good about myself, I feel normal . . . my clothes fit better and I can wear the same blouses that I had [before the surgery] . . . when I wore a C cup. . . . I feel comfortable in my clothes." While Rachel's comfort came from a restored sense of comfort in her clothes, lost temporarily to mastectomy surgery, Ashley's security was new. Reflecting on her experiences before implant surgery, Ashley compared her new level of confidence with an old anxious memory:

> It was so nice after I had my surgery. [When playing] . . . beach volleyball . . . it was so nice to be able to raise both arms up to hit the ball and my bathing suit stay in place and not come up to my shoulders which is what would basically happen [before the implants]. Like when you raise your [arms], your shirt may come up on your stomach when you stretch. It's almost the same thing but when your swimsuit comes up above your chest. . . . It is that bad.

Now more fully endowed, Ashley's swimsuit remained over her breasts when she played sports.

Swimsuits continued to be important elements in postimplant stories. Julia told her surgeon "I want simply the smallest implant I can get; just enough to fill out my swimsuit top." Ashley found shopping for a swimsuit to be a much more enjoyable experience: "Oh, it's been, I mean it's been great. . . . In a store, I can find a bra that fits me. I can find a swimsuit that fits me and bottoms are the same size, you know, and whereas before, I would have to go to a specialty shop and buy like a much smaller top than a bottom, and so that aspect has been great."

Freedom.   Very few of the women reported dressing provocatively after their implant surgery. Several indicated that the operation had not changed their dress at all. Elaine's husband told her he was perplexed by the fact that she still hid her nice figure under baggy tops. Yet, for many women, the implants allowed them to experiment with different kinds of clothing they had been too concerned to wear in the past.

Most women reported being able to relax about their clothing, "It was such a freedom when I had the implants the first time to be able to wear what I wanted to wear." For most women, the experimentation with clothes was minor. Julia said, "I dress a little more sexy . . . a little less conservatively." Pat expressed one of the small but significant advantages of the implants: "I can go now without a bra unless I have something see-through, I don't have to wear a bra."

Other women were more adventuresome. Marie's "after implant" story included a new found-freedom in dress. Before the implants, she "would purposely look for a type of lingerie that was maybe gathered across the bust line." She explained that she "really wasn't comfortable lounging around in any type of thing like that without my bra because it emphasized the flatness there." After her implants, she reported having a great time at the lingerie store:

I really did. It was wonderful to be able to go to the rack that was not padded and to be able to, you know, all the little matching outfits. . . . Well, they don't make those for padded bras. . . . So it was fun. . . . My husband had been in San Francisco . . . and he went to Victoria's Secret. . . . And he came back with all these wonderful little matching things. And I enjoyed all that for a while. It got old, you know. Right now, I'm into comfort. You know, cotton panties, something like that. But it was nice . . . to have that option, and I really enjoyed it.

Small freedoms in clothing are significant for the women we talked to. Julia explained that her changes in clothing following the implants were minimal, but she "didn't mind wearing a tight blouse as much" as she did before. Ashley estimated that her camouflaging techniques, "choosing blousey" clothing to conceal her flat chest, were not as important after the implants.

The differences in women before and after their implants were not usually major, but almost always positive. They uniformly felt more self-confident, less self-conscious, and more relaxed about their dress. It is important to note that these positive results were not limited to the women who were satisfied with their implants. Even women who linked grave illnesses to their implants also reported significant benefits to their implants. Convinced that her implants were threatening her life, Toni still recalled their benefits:

Most of the women that I talked to, that had implants, that are not in the ill period, really enjoy the implant decision. And they feel good about it. Everybody throughout their whole life is searching to put their self-esteem in a good place, and they [implants] . . . can be one of the accessories in life to help a woman get, get her self-esteem in an undamaged state.

For Toni, and other women who were sick, the illness overshadowed the benefits, but the blow to self-esteem from implant removal was great: "When they start getting ill, that changes and a lot of them, when they first start getting the idea that there is a connection, it's a very difficult decision to give up that part of their body and their life and their self-image. It's a very big, damaging bite."

One difference in the sick women's stories and the satisfied women's stories was the perception of benefits and risks. Linking their grave illnesses to the implants, the sick women judged their implants not worth the problems related to them. Satisfied women also reported experiencing health problems but they were not as numerous, not perceived to be as serious, or not linked to the implants.

WOMEN'S PHYSICAL EXPERIENCE WITH IMPLANTS

Initially it is important to note that the women who were satisfied with their implants reported a much smaller number of problems. Notably, they had fewer ruptures and replacements. Of the 20 women linking illnesses to their implants, seven required no replacements, five required one replacement, and six women required two replacements. One sick woman had four sets before she finally had the implants removed permanently. In comparison, most of the satisfied women had not experienced ruptures, leakage, or replacements. Twelve of the 15 women still had their original set of implants. Two of the women had their implants replaced once. One woman was on her third set.

The satisfied women reported very positive physical experiences—"no scars"—the implants were "perfect." Most indicated that their implants looked good. Several commented that their implants were soft; they had experienced no hardening. Most reported they would "do it again" and were "very satisfied."

Nonetheless, women who were happy with their implants were not free of problems. Their stories included multiple health and aesthetic problems following their implant surgery: asymmetrical placement, painful breasts, unnatural looking breast separation, breast numbness, capsular contraction, keloiding, inability to breast feed, arthritis, unexplained joint pain, heart problems, rashes, intense chest pressure, swelling, gall bladder problems, and edema. However, in their stories about health, the satisfied women told fewer stories about problems than did the sick women, minimized the problems, and/or did not link their difficulties to their implants.

When talking about their implant surgery and subsequent problems, many women mentioned problems briefly and then appeared to dismiss them as unimportant. Irene described her implant surgery in which she "lost a lot of blood and was very, very weak." Despite these difficulties, she balanced the problems with other things that went well. "I had lymph nodes out, but I had not really had any swelling in my arms." The evaluation she drew on balance was that, "I had no trouble with my surgery . . . I had a wonderful recovery." She continued, explaining, "I have some discomfort sometimes, but, you know, not anything . . . that I can't live with."

This pattern is repeated in Janine's description of painful sensitivity in her nipples, following surgery. She notes the problems, but minimizes them, evaluating the whole experience as positive:

> I haven't had any problem other than the sensitivity is greatly increased. It's almost painful sometimes around the nipple area. Like to touch, which I never had that before, but other than that I don't have a problem. It almost hurts, they are very, very sore, but it's just around the nipple area, the rest of it is just fine.

A positive overall evaluation of the implants occurs frequently when women admit they have problems but judge them as less negative than their situation before the implants. According to Rachel, her surgery was "less painful than a biopsy." Elizabeth was willing to swap "some numbness" in her breasts for "peace of mind" knowing that she was not at risk for breast cancer. She reasoned that the lack of sensitivity in her breasts "didn't really bother me because it's not like a limb that you use everyday." Marie wished her breasts looked "a little more real or something. . . . There seems to be a definite separation, if you look at them at the right angle. And there seems to be an unnatural type of curve at the top." She concluded, however, "I'm just not going to complain." She found the implants, unnatural as they looked, to be much preferable to her previously small breasts. "It's just so much better than what was there. Absolutely."

Minimization of difficulties also occurred when women explained that the problems were expected. A plastic surgeon or friend had warned them ahead of time. Frances experienced hardening in her first two sets of implants and clammy, chilled skin in the breast area. She accepted the problems as normal because her plastic surgeon had explained the symptom as just part of the "implant process." Julia's implants sagged following the birth of her child. Although she was disappointed, she explained that her physician had told her ahead of time that her implants might not be as perfect as other women she knew; that experiences differed due to variations in chest muscles and elasticity. Elizabeth's friends had forewarned her about possible loss of breast sensation.

In addition, the satisfied women seldom related health problems to their implants, linking them instead to other causes. Both Frances and Gillian suffered from arthritis, but neither believed the pain was caused by implants. Frances explained that arthritis ran in her family. Julia blamed her sagging implants on pregnancy and breast feeding. Amy related her shrunken implants to severe weight loss. Rachel's swelling and edema were blamed on the removal of lymph nodes. Marie explained that a "heavy sense of pressure in her chest . . . almost panic" was a result of her personality:

> Of course, I am panic-prone anyway. And I know the first time [I] had them [implants], I felt like someone had set a concrete block on my chest and I began to hyperventilate and I really had to work with myself to relax, you know, and to breath properly. . . . I would have to, you know, take deep breaths and to basically practice the same type of things that I would practice when I would be on a plane and begin to feel claustrophobic.

As a rule, the satisfied women did not believe that their health problems were attributable to their implants, even when their symptoms were similar to the problems that the sick women related to silicone. Gillian's explanation is typical of satisfied women's attitudes about illness and implants. As she prepared to replace ruptured implants with another pair filled with silicone gel, Gillian discounted links between her arthritis pain and her implants:

> I do have problems with [arthritis]. Wouldn't it be wonderful if these [implants] all came out and they cleaned up the capsule and threw some more in and 6 months later I don't have as much arthritis? Wouldn't that be great? But, I don't expect that. I think that's whistling in the dark.

Most of the satisfied women we talked to explicitly stated that they had experienced "no problems" with their implants; among those were Rachel, Janine,

Patricia, Irene, Elizabeth, Lorraine, Marie, Leanne, and Gillian. Yet in their postimplant surgery stories, all these women also described complications: hardening, swelling, pain, breast separation, ruptures, arthritis, and edema. The women's tendency to discount these problems is highlighted in Gillian's connection between attitudes and health problems:

> I really feel your experience depends upon your personal attitude and your view of yourself and your body and who you are. I don't know, I just feel if you are happy with yourself and happy with who you are, you just kind of do it. You accept what has to be done and you do it and if things don't come out quite right, which of course mine [implants] are not symmetrical, one's a little hard and one's a little soft, its just no big deal—they are there. It's my preference they be there than nothing be there. I don't want to wear [a prosthesis] in my bra and I think you make that decision and that's the way you want to go, then put it on a shelf and forget it.

We found it notable that the satisfied women so consistently excused the implants and characterized problems as "no big deal." One explanation for their attitudes can be found in their discussion of health risks.

AWARENESS OF HEALTH RISKS
ASSOCIATED WITH BREAST IMPLANTS

News about health risks associated with breasts implants came to the satisfied women not from their own experiences, nor from their friends and physicians, but from news media. The reports of connective tissues disease, rashes, infections, and other illnesses came as a surprise. Almost all the satisfied women knew others who were having good experiences with their implants. The majority of their friends were "very pleased." Marie's acquaintances were "very happy." A dear friend of Irene's had silicone implants for 26 years. Irene reported, "She's fine." Of Janine's friends, "none had problems." One of Leanne's clients had silicone implants but was "not having problems." When asked about health problems, Ashley replied that risks "don't concern me." She explained, "I don't know anyone . . . that has had a problem with it [implants], so it's hard for me to relate [to women who are having problems] hypothetically." Like Ashley, most satisfied women knew few, if any, friends experiencing difficulties with the devices. Of the few who knew women having problems, most of our interviewees doubted that their ailments were caused by silicone.

It was, instead, the media that served as the messenger of danger. We asked Janine about the source of her concern regarding safety. She replied, "Probably just the media. At that time [when she got the implants], I did not know anyone who had any problems with it." Elaine explained the impact of news coverage. She worked in a medical office, and following the *Connie Chung* program, "The unit was getting so many calls those days about implants, and everyone was like

'AHHH!' Up in their arms about it." Patricia indicated that she had "only" received information about implant problems from television. "I think it's probably normal for the media. Anything that happens they are going to blow it up and make a story out of it."

Most of the satisfied women said they either ignored the media accounts or considered them biased sources of information. If they watched the controversy carefully, they interpreted the accounts with skepticism. Patricia's reaction to the reports was, "I am not really a worrier, so why should I worry about this until something [occurs]. I had no reason." Julia explained that she "was blowing it off," paying little attention to news accounts until recently. Irene purposefully ignored the reports:

> I chose not to read about any of it because I had decided that I'm going to keep mine. It's just like I don't read a lot of articles about breast cancer because I've had my breasts removed. . . . And I could just sit around, you know, worrying about every little, teeny, tiny thing, and maybe that's being a little bit of an ostrich but I just feel like, I have no reason to believe at this point that I'm not as cured as I possibly can be and I'm very satisfied with my implants. . . . I've stopped reading about that because, you know, you can just scare yourself to death.

Most of those who followed the news characterized the coverage as biased against implants. Rachel explained, "I really don't think much of the media, so I'm prejudiced." Frances believed that the media have "blown the controversy out of proportion" and wondered why the press did not do a background health check on women who were reporting problems. Several characterized the "sensationalist" tendencies of the media as creating a bigger problem than existed: "There are a lot more satisfied women with implants than there are dissatisfied ones. . . . We're talking about a few hundred [women]." According to Janine, the news bias occurred because "the only ones [women] you see [on the news] are the ones having problems. Getting the people who are not having problems to come forth or talk about it, people just aren't going to do that."

Some satisfied women did not pay attention to the news because they had saline implants and they felt that the accounts of danger did not apply to them. When we asked her if she had heard any news about problems with implants, Elaine answered, "Some, you know, but it's more with the silicone. It doesn't really pertain to me that much." Like Elaine, Marie felt immune to the news because her implants were saline. "I didn't follow up on it [the media] enough. . . . I'm sure that if I had silicone, I would be following it to this day!" But several with silicone implants discounted the media reports as well. Ashley, who had her silicone implants for 5 years, called the news "media hype" and paid little attention: "I am not one to read the newspapers, so I know I missed a lot of it. But I . . . know how media hype is, just from working in where I work . . . just how distorted the stories are. I know firsthand how that can be, so I take it with a grain of salt."

Lorraine concurred, explaining that news media tend toward negative accounts: "The media looks at the bad things rather than the good. . . . That's led to . . . a few . . . of these doctors and . . . some people [who] like to cause controversial things like that."

As women talked about the implant-related illnesses covered in the press, they revealed attitudes about health care and risk in general. Most of the satisfied women attributed the sick women's ailments, like their own health problems, to causes other than the implants. Elaine speculated, "Perhaps they just had something in their genetic histories that this has triggered." Irene attributed one woman's implant problems to stress. Janine blamed the complicated and vague symptoms on aging:

I think some of the problems could be psychological. I think women between the ages of 30 to 55 are experiencing all sorts of changes in their body, not only physical but emotional and sometimes they want a reason or excuse for some of the fatigue and aches and pains and changes in their body. I am not so sure that it's all attributed to silicone implants.

Several others, besides Elaine, linked the ailments to emotional disturbance. Rachel explained:

The only complaints they have had from the silicone breast and the breast implants have been primarily with women who wanted the enhancement. . . . The women, the ones who have, were having emotional problems and needed the enhancements. [They] were the ones that were complaining. At the time [I got my implants], they felt that there was no greater number of complaints from the silicone breast implants than there was a normal number of those picking up Lupus or rheumatoid arthritis or scleroderma or any of the other diseases. . . . I thought it was rather interesting because you're dealing with a personality and not just a physical complaint.

Gillian concurred with Rachel's characterization as she described Jenny Jones' complaints about her implants as "hysterical." Irene used the same term to describe her sister's concern over her implants.

As they wondered about the causes for sick women's problems, our interviewees revealed strong beliefs that individual variations among patients cause different outcomes of medical procedures and that health decisions are inherently risky. Rachel said, "There is no product that is foreign to the body that can be taken without a side effect. . . . You look into all these other things . . . not just breast implants . . . [For example], I get migraine headaches from Nutrasweet." Irene and Rachel, both doctor's wives, attributed implant problems to the fact that different people have a variety of reactions to the same medical procedure. Irene explained, "I mean if you go and have your toe removed, there's a few people that, you know, 30 people have their toes removed, there are a few of them that won't do real well."

Several women focused on the normally expected risks inherent in surgery and any kind of implanted device: "Anytime you, you anticipate surgery, anytime you put a foreign body in, you're going to get some kind of rejection. You're going to get an inflammatory reaction, you're going to get side effects." Lorraine and Amy compared the possibility of rejecting implants to the risks of heart and lung transplants. According to Lorraine:

> Any time you have something replaced in your body, whether it's a kidney implant or a heart implant or whatever it may be, you stand a chance, you stand the chance of rejecting [it]. . . . I don't see any difference in breast implants; you still stand the chance of rejecting those just like you do anything else. . . . These women, there's no doubt in my mind that [they] may . . . be having these problems. They are just like people that can't accept a heart transplant or a kidney transplant or whatever other transplants they may have to have.

Although most satisfied women were not sure why other women were having problems, they speculated that the sick women suffered from illnesses unrelated to their implants and characterized the problems as heightened by psychological disturbances. Many believed that if silicone implants did cause problems, the risks were normal, comparable to other medical procedures, and not unique to silicone implants.

Not all the satisfied women shared the view that silicone was not a special threat. Even the majority, who held reassuring opinions of silicone's general safety, made occasional statements that revealed lingering concern about the risks, which they had heard about in the news. A few women perceived the media coverage of implant problems to have created an important public awareness of potential problems. Elizabeth praised the news reports, "I think it's [media coverage] good. I think it's showing both sides." Leanne credited the accounts with bringing previously hidden problems "to people's attention."

Elizabeth and Leanne acted on the news of risks, choosing saline implants rather than silicone because they believed that silicone was dangerous. According to Leanne, "The minute all this really came out in the media . . . I had every intention of doing silicone." After her physician told Leanne that the aesthetic affect of saline was the same as for silicone, she opted for the noncontroversial implant.

Only Leanne and Elizabeth purposefully gathered information from media that conclusively decided the type of implants they chose. However, several others who had implants after 1990 also rejected silicone. Even though they were unconvinced that silicone posed a definite and unique threat, they chose saline because it was "uncontroversial." Rachel "eliminated any kind of the silicone implants because they were controversial." Janine also chose saline: "My feeling is, if there is a lot of controversy, I would rather be safe than sorry down the road, you know."

Some of those who chose saline over silicone drew a clear difference between saline's natural characteristics and silicone's "foreign" threat. Saline was described as "natural" and safe. If it deflates, there is no problem. Elizabeth explained her choice on the basis of possible leaks:

I'm trying to hurdle past getting cancer . . . I don't want anything else to happen to me. To worry about, "Gee, what if it leaks?" . . . I'm going to have these for the rest of my life. I don't want anything breaking in me that's going to release anything toxic in my system. You know, if it's salt water, fine. It'll just be absorbed.

Elaine's characterization of silicone was similar:

I didn't want to have to worry about possible leakage, but it was my choice, the saline. . . . Just having a foreign body in your system, [silicone] is a little bit kind of scary to begin with too, so that was, I think, my major thing. I didn't want my system to go out of whack.

Silicone was characterized by several women who recently chose saline implants, with the potential to poison or distress the body. The characterization sounded very much like the descriptions of sick women from previous chapters.

Although most of the satisfied women did not believe that silicone posed a danger, we noticed ambivalence in their comments. Within a single interview, a woman would discount the implant-related illnesses as psychological or attribute them to other causes. A few minutes later, the same woman described choices she made that were founded in the possibility of silicone danger. Janine described the media as negatively biased and attributed a friend's implant problems to bad rapport with her plastic surgeon. Yet, Janine chose saline over silicone. Patricia remarked that she would recommend silicone implants to her daughter. "I have no reason not to. I don't think there has been any real proof has there?" Yet, she monitors her movements to prevent leakage. "I am very careful. . . . I wouldn't deliberately bump into anything, but I am careful. I don't sleep on my stomach anymore. I sleep on my side." Amy doesn't know what to think. She is experiencing no problems herself and completely ignored media reports. Recently, however, her sister and mother have experienced new rashes and allergies. She "flip-flops back and forth" about safety. She recalled that she's had a number of migraine headaches recently. She's "not sure when they started." But "you hear so many symptoms" related to the illness; it makes her wonder.

Few of the satisfied women were without some doubt about the safety of implants, particularly about silicone. Rachel and Amy expressed concern about even "the little bit of silicone" they have in the shell of their saline implants. Only Irene appeared to have no doubts about the safety of the implants. Only Elizabeth and Leanne seemed completely convinced that silicone is dangerous. All the others fell somewhere in between. They conveyed a sense of confidence that they were not at risk for implant-related illnesses. Just as clearly, media accounts of implant risks have planted a small seed of concern.

IMPLICATIONS

Some elements of the satisfied women's collective stories struck us as particularly noteworthy, both in their differences and similarities to the sick women's narratives. Unlike accounts described in earlier chapters, the satisfied women's accounts had few villains. For both groups of women, the relationship with their physicians seemed important in the way they experienced their health care. Expectations about health played a significant role in both sets of narratives, but the expectations were different. Influences outside the medical community played equally important roles in the narratives of the sick and satisfied women. For both groups, the women's sense of femininity and self-esteem was closely connected to their breasts.

Unlike the narratives of the sick women, the satisfied women had less need and less tendency to vilify their physicians. An obvious reason might be that the satisfied women had fewer health problems and so less need to find a reason for them (including blaming others). A less obvious reason was revealed in attitudes expressed by the satisfied women regarding control over medical outcomes. The satisfied women characterized health decisions as inherently risky, outside of the realm of human control. Their statements comparing complications of breast implants describe medical risks as ever present. More relaxed attitudes toward implant problems, accepting complications as "no big deal" or "no problem," are characteristic of individuals with less need for control (Crawford, 1984).

An important manifestation of the satisfied woman's different attitude was her reaction to mistakes made by the doctors. Like the sick women, many of the satisfied women were originally told that the devices would last forever. In retrospect, all the women we talked to perceived that ruptures and leaks were the norm rather than the exception. The satisfied women who experienced leaks, ruptures, and deflations characterized the early reassurances as human error and the "state of the art" at the time rather than as malicious betrayal by the medical community.

Gillian's reaction to ruptures in her silicone implants is a good example of the satisfied women's recognition of physician error. Although she suspected that a radiologist who was "not careful" when taking a mammogram caused a rupture, Gillian was philosophic and forgiving when discussing her need for replacements:

> They told me in '77, "This [implant] is going to last forever." I didn't question it any further. It didn't dawn on me to question it further, but I do remember them saying that, because I had a good rapport with the doctor. The doctor that I had was the head of plastic surgery at Duke at that time, Dr. X, you know, he just laughed about it. And I said, "You mean when I die they are still going to be there?" And he said, "You are going to be laid out, they are still going to be up there." I mean, that was their attitude at that time. And of course they were mistaken. But I don't have any, I don't know. It was an error, nothing in our bodies last. A hip replacement is silicone, it doesn't last. . . . And if there was an error. It was yes, they did think it was a lifelong entity.

Gillian's blameless acceptance of her physician's mistakes is more characteristic of the satisfied women, who, like Irene, said of their doctors, "They are not God." This acceptance could be the result of the more positive relationship described in the satisfied women's accounts regarding doctor–patient rapport. In these narratives, the physicians are a primary source of control and support, helpful in healing (Brody, 1987). Focusing primarily on the plastic surgeons, the satisfied women portray them as agents who facilitated problem solving. Through the skill of their surgeons, the women overcame fears of breast cancer, the painful anxiety of fibrocystic disease, and years of low self-esteem.

In addition, the plastic surgeons were portrayed as a major source of support. The women, who chose the plastic surgeons they had known for years or had performed previous medical operations for them, had proof of the doctors' sustained interest in their health. Other women told stories about doctors who spent significant amounts of time with their patients, provided ongoing access to them, and communicated caring through various follow-up procedures. Unlike the sick women whose doctor–patient stories included abandonment and rejection, most of the satisfied women perceived a solid foundation of support and trust in their plastic surgeons.

The importance of a positive doctor–patient relationship to health is recognized, not only by scholars, but by the women themselves. When Janine was describing the only woman she knew who was having problems with her implants, she described a situation founded in a poor relationship between the patient and her plastic surgeon.

> The doctor never . . . he never answered, he never really told her much. But she didn't ask any questions. . . . I think she felt very intimidated to ask any questions. . . . This girl walked out of there with nothing. . . . The doctor didn't offer her anything. . . . No pamphlets whatsoever. No information.

Good rapport with a trusted physician seems to have played a major role in the satisfaction of women with breast implants.

Comparisons between the two groups of women and their different relationships with physicians is complicated by a major variation in narrative time. Most satisfied women told stories about encounters with physicians early in the implant experience. Sick women focused on interactions with doctors much later, in some cases, years after the initial implant surgery. When asked about earlier experiences, many women who blamed illness on their implants did not provide much, if any, detail. The salient narrative issues in the sick women's stories focused on encounters with physicians after the onset of disease.

In addition to different doctor–patient relationships, alternate expectations contributed to the difference in the stories represented by the sick women and the satisfied women. The narratives provide different frameworks for interpreting physical experiences. In both sets of stories, the women relied on social networks to understand their experiences with breast implants. The sick women told stories about recognizing themselves in the accounts of dissatisfied women in news reports and support groups. Through identification with those stories, the sick women found diagnoses, guidance, and coping strategies. The satisfied women had equally influential social support that provided guidance, but the network was composed of women with good implant experiences. Further, their extensive effort to find out about implants before their decisions to have the surgery, put them in touch with other women who had good implant experiences.

Many of the satisfied women we talked to were connected with one another. Two thirds of our interviewees knew someone else we interviewed; several sets were relatives. One third of the satisfied women were related to physicians or were employed in the medical profession. The mirrors that the satisfied women used for reflection, interpretation, and identification were other satisfied women and a group that was closely associated with the medical community.

Such a group was less likely to blame physicians or to focus on negative experiences. According to Brody (1987), "Stories serve to relate individual experiences to the explanatory constructs of the society and culture and also to place the experiences within the context of a particular individual's life history" (p. 5). For the satisfied women, their experience with implants was placed within the context of other women who perceived their implant complications to be inconveniences or related to other causes. The group reinforced individual positive attitudes.

The ability to place illness and problems into one's belief system and life history may also have played a role in the more positive experiences of the satisfied women. The sick women's stories were characterized by an inability to relate illness to life previous to the implants. The satisfied women, however, were often able to integrate implant and other health problems within a coherent story. Frances' arthritis was not a mystery; she related it to a family history with the illness. Marie's chest pressure fit into her sense of identity, "I am panic prone." To her, it was a familiar, if uncomfortable, feeling similar to the panic attacks she had on airplanes. Irene's sister's concern about her implants was consistent with a "hysterical" personality.

Implant problems were integrated as well into the story of implants that the women received from their plastic surgeons and their friends. Ashley's implants hardened because she did not do the exercises her doctor said would prevent encapsulation. Elizabeth was prepared for numbness in her breasts following surgery because her friends with implants told her that might occur. The satisfied women had contexts in which to place their ailments and experiences. The sick women did not. Different expectations appear to have made a difference in the stories the two sets of women tell about their implants.

The importance of influences beyond the medical community in women's health care decisions is clear in both group's accounts. Even though most satisfied women trusted and respected their physicians, they all relied on other sources of health information and most were influenced, to some degree, by media accounts of health risks. Whereas sick women reported a reliance on self-help groups and the media, family was critical in the satisfied women's stories.

The impact of family medical history is particularly notable for the women whose relatives had a high level of breast cancer and fibrocystic disease. The women whose family members died of breast cancer were convinced that, unless they acted, they also would contract the disease. Several resisted their physicians' advice against preventive mastectomies.

Equally apparent was the influence of family members on the acceptability of implant procedures. About one half of the satisfied women had family members who also had implants. Several were mother–daughter or sister combinations. Close knowledge of another person's experience with implants is likely to make the procedure more acceptable and to build a framework for setting expectations. When combined with the fact that almost all the satisfied women had close friends who had implants, it is clear that most group members had a positive context for interpreting their implant experience.

Of all the commonalities between the sick and the satisfied women's stories, the one that surprised us most was the absence of men in the narratives. We expected to hear motivation stories that included male partners. We expected that women would talk about a desire to attract mates or to increase sexual appeal. Those stories were almost entirely absent. Only Patricia reported that she had implants to please a significant other. The overwhelming response in motivation was, "I did it for myself."

When we asked women about the affect that the implants had on their relationships with significant others, the response was minimal. Most of the women were married at the time they had their implants; a few were engaged to be married. Rachel was recently widowed, indicating that having implants to attract men "was not a high priority." Women did not have the implants to attract mates; most already had significant relationships.

Several women indicated that they had not even discussed the implant decision with their partner. Amy said that she announced her decision to her fiancé , and he replied, "Do you need a ride to the doctor's office?" Women characterized their husbands as supportive of them, regardless of their chest size or physical appearance. As Elaine talked about her husband, she concluded, "I have a wonderful man who loves me no matter if I had one arm and one leg. I mean he was very happy with me. It's what's inside me."

Women claimed responsibility for their decision to have breast implants: "You want to do it, then you do it, but you do it for yourself. You don't do it because someone wants you to or whatever; you have to be happy with yourself. You have to be happy with yourself inside first and like yourself to begin with."

Although women said that men were not their motivation, several reported that the implants had improved the relationships they had with their partners. The increased intimacy had less to do with the men, however, than the internal changes perceived by these women. Ashley credited the changes to increased self-esteem, "It made a difference in my sexual life . . . my self-esteem . . . That made such a big difference." Marie concurred. Her implants allowed her to be less self-conscious and more comfortable with her husband:

I felt more comfortable. I felt like I could be more relaxed. Of course, I didn't have to deal with multiple partners. It was just my husband. But, and I didn't feel a sense of self-consciousness about it. It took me a while to get used to, you know, having breasts. But it wasn't like I was trying to fool him. You know, he knew that they weren't real. And they just . . . I became more aware of my body in many ways. But then less concerned with it. I wasn't preoccupied with how I look right now, you know. Or of trying to wear something that didn't emphasize my breasts. And I just . . . it really helped me to relax in that regard.

Self-esteem and comfort with one's body are significant benefits for all the women we interviewed. Regardless of the motive or the result of implant surgery, breasts were perceived by almost all women, sick and satisfied, to be important to their sense of femininity and wholeness. Both the sick and the satisfied women's stories confirm the vital connection between the women's bodies and their sense of self-worth and identity.

Many women we talked to connected their gender identity and their self-esteem to their appearance. When the body failed to conform to the expected norm, regardless of the reason, women felt inadequate or uncomfortable. These feelings affected a wide variety of the women's lives. The women's stories confirm Natanson's (1970) declaration, "I am neither 'in' my body nor 'attached to' it; it does not belong to me or go along with me. *I am my body*" (p. 12). This statement may be particularly true in the relationship between women and their breasts. "How could her breasts fail to be an aspect of her identity, since they emerge for [a woman] at that time in her life when her sense of her own independent identity is finally formed? For many women, if not all, breasts are an important component of body self-image" (Young, 1990, p. 189). Physicians treating women with breast implants are dealing with far more than lumps of fatty tissue; they are treating the patient's sense of self.

5

DOCTORS IN CONFLICT: DIFFERENT SPECIALTIES, DIFFERENT STORIES

INTRODUCTION: PROBLEM AND METHOD

As our interest in the silicone gel breast implant controversy grew, we began to talk to some of the doctors involved. We had become interested initially because two plastic surgeons wanted our advice. We had talked with them at length. As we sought patients to interview, we began an informal dialogue with a rheumatologist. It was clear from the outset that these physicians differed in what they saw happening to patients. Because patients look to physicians to interpret both the scientific information and the patients' own experiences, the views of physicians are essential in understanding this controversy; both how the uncertainty and contradictions have developed and how they have affected patients.

Our study of the press coverage reported in chapter 6 found doctors disagreeing. A local press conference featured a plastic surgeon and a rheumatologist presenting inconsistent views and advice. Print journalists balanced their stories of patient problems often by eliciting comments from doctors of differing opinions. The popular view of doctors as a monolithic guild, protecting each other by masking disagreements, must have been shaken by these clashes of physicians' opinion regarding implants. Doctors presented contradictory evidence and judgments quite openly.

Privately, they criticized each other as well. Terms like "greed," "junk science," and "plastic men" occasionally peppered their comments when we talked to them. During the heat of the controversy, three plastic surgeons filed a formal complaint with the Florida Department of Professional Regulation alleging that one rheumatologist had used shoddy diagnostic practices, told women they had diseases that did not exist, and solicited patients unethically. Here was clearly a case where we could examine differences of opinion within the medical community.

We had been interested for some time in the general question of how patients and the public act when information about health appears uncertain, unclear, and/or contradictory. The implant controversy increasingly became a dramatic case of such information ambiguity. How, we wondered, could doctors have such strong and contradictory opinions and advice? If the scientific evidence was not clear, would they not speak with more caution and sound more open to the views of those who differed? If doctors traditionally are reluctant to question others openly, what was different here? We began to think that we were in the middle of a case that might teach us about communication and the formation of opinion within the medical community.

We, thus, began a series of interviews with doctors whose women patients were likely to ask about implants, but whose specialties differed. We pursued the following research questions:

1. How do physicians view implant patients and their experiences?
2. How do they view the efficacy of implants?
3. How do they view the scientific evidence about implant safety?
4. Do their answers differ along specialty lines?

To answer these questions, we interviewed 14 doctors: 3 rheumatologists, 6 plastic surgeons, 1 general surgeon, 1 family physician, and 3 obstetrician/gynecologists. One rheumatologist had been prominently involved, appearing before the FDA and Congress on this issue. One plastic surgeon had been an advisor to the FDA on implant safety. Three of the interviewees were female: a plastic surgeon, a gynecologist, and a family physician.

The interviews were scheduled in the physicians' offices. A consent form was signed and the doctors were assured of confidentiality. No records of the physicians' names were kept. Most interviews lasted 45 to 60 minutes. Interviews were audio recorded and transcribed. The interview schedule appears as Fig. 5.1. The analysis presented later was done from the transcripts. Interviews were open ended. Most questions on the schedule were asked of most doctors, but the interviewees were encouraged to follow their own ideas and agendas. They were asked to give stories and examples throughout to illustrate the general points they were making.

In the interviews, we began with the same attention to narrative we had used to look at the stories of patients. We sought stories, but not all the doctors were good storytellers. On some topics, in particular, they appeared to be more comfortable in abstract discourse. Probing for examples yielded only further exposition, not narration. Our analysis began by looking for narrative themes, and we found some, but to be true to the nature of the doctor's responses, we also reflect their abstractions as well. Consequently, although our report uses physicians' stories for illustration, the pattern of topics derives as much from the nature of the questions asked as from physicians' narratives.

We report on what physicians told us in four sections corresponding to the four research questions: patient experiences, implant efficacy, implant safety and science, and specialty differences.

1. What experience have you had with patients involved with silicone breast implants?
2. How did you first become involved with this problem?
3. What did you think about it at first? How has your understanding developed?
4. What are typical patients' reasons for seeing you about implants? Do you think their reasons for seeing you are good ones?
5. Do you think that the women who have had implants have done so for good reasons?
6. What are some examples of the patient stories you hear?
7. There has been some controversy about the use of implants.
   a. What do you understand the problems to be that have generated this controversy?
   b. Do you think implants are safe?
   c. What scientific evidence convinces you that that view is correct?
   d. Not all physicians have the same view of the evidence. How do you regard the arguments of those who see the evidence differently? Are they being scientific? What is necessary for appropriate science to fit this problem?
   e. What motivates those who see the issues differently?
   f. Some of the difference of opinion among doctors seems to fall along specialty lines. How do you see this difference in approach from the different specialties? How should patients react when they get different advice from different doctors?
8. A number of women have been outspokenly critical of doctors who have performed implants and of manufacturers of implants? Have these women behaved appropriately?
9. Some women who have had breasts removed due to cancer have argued that silicone implants are absolutely essential. How do you respond to their views?
10. Has the press treated the issues appropriately?
11. Has the FDA acted properly? If not, what should they have done differently?
12. Have the implant manufacturers behaved properly? If not, what should they have done differently?
13. If we could look back on this question from some point in the future when the issue was behind us, what do you suppose we will find the true story to be?

FIG. 5.1. Physicians interview schedule re: silicone breast implants.

PATIENTS AND THEIR EXPERIENCES

Doctor Reports of Patient Stories

The interviews reported here are with doctors, not with patients, but the doctors did talk about their patients. They often reported what their patients had told them about experiences with their implants, with symptoms, and with other doctors. It is important to remember that the descriptions of patient experiences come from the doctors and, consequently, are secondhand, not first person accounts. Nonetheless, they are consistent with the stories we heard from the women we interviewed.

As in all aspects of this study, the stories about patients with problems are the most dramatic, but it is important to remember that they are not typical of most women who have had implants. In our media study reported in chapter 6, we found that the press coverage featured the stories of the women with problems and paid comparatively little attention to the women whose experiences were positive. In our survey, (see chap. 9) women with implants were overwhelmingly positive about them. In our interviews, some doctors also talked about patients with positive experiences.

Early in his career, a plastic surgeon explained he had been reluctant to put in implants. He had not been sure they were really needed for reasons other than vanity:

> After a couple of years . . . I began to see patients like a young lady who was 19, who would literally become terrified when someone would whisper the word "beach" to her because of the idea of getting into a bathing suit and showing an almost scaphoid chest. She was so embarrassed. This girl was a social cripple. I put a set of breasts in her, which have been no problem to her; not large, just a normal set of breasts and that young lady not only went to the beach, but in a few years she was married and has been a very happy person. That fearful, anxious look that she had even when we weren't talking about the beach is gone now. This is just an example of a person who really needed augmentation.

Clearly, in this story the woman had a positive outcome with her breast implants. The story is one of success. It has a happy ending. The woman is portrayed as someone who is easy to identify with. She was self-conscious for good reasons and has been helped by her physician's skill and the availability of an effective medical device.

A family physician talked about one of her patients:

> She had had two or three children and breast fed and her breasts were very flat. Her husband found it a turn off so she'd had implants put in and that had been quite successful. . . . I'm sure there was a kernel of discomfort with the news in the press, but, on the other hand, she herself had not experienced any problems from the implants.

The women who have had difficulties do have compelling experiences, however. The rheumatologists we interviewed saw implant patients only when they were experiencing rheumatic symptoms. One described this group of patients:

Most of these women who get implants are . . . upscale women. Most of the time it's done for purely cosmetic reasons. . . . Insurance won't pay. They have good jobs and they're bright. And, you know, they get tired and they can tell. . . . It's so insidious that they're 35 years old and they're supposed to be tired. They have three kids or six kids and they're supposed to be tired. They fool themselves for a while. Some of them are very tolerant of their symptoms, but at some point they know this isn't right. They go to their plastic surgeons or their primary care doctors who tell them, "It's menopause," or "It's depression," or "It's getting older," or some nebuloma. Either they accept it—and I'm sure a lot of them accepted what the physician told them—but a lot of them know they're sick. They run from physician to physician to physician trying to get an answer. Eventually some of them ran into me . . . and I said, "Could be the implants." Most of them don't jump for joy or anything. Most of them have a very tough decision about whether to remove the implants or not.

Another rheumatologist portrayed implant patients as follows:

I've seen some women who have gotten implants at an early age, like in their mid-20s. . . . They were working hard and were really going in the right direction and who became sick after their implants. This was long before there was any publicity. They bring with them records where they've gone to infectious disease specialists, rheumatologists . . . psychiatrists. They've been to all kinds of people . . . I've seen women whose entire lives have changed after the implants.

A large number of these women really have gone through a tremendously terrible experience because of just the mechanical problems of the implants. They've had repeated operations. The silicone implants have burst. They've caused erosions of the skin. They've drained. They've given chest wall pain. Some of these women have really had a nightmare, a nightmare over a decade with their silicone implants . . . necrotic tissue, capsulization with pain, deformity.

The narratives of such patients' experiences have been moving to their doctors. They are moving to us, as we hear them even second- and thirdhand. None of the doctors we interviewed doubted that some women were having great difficulties, only whether their implants were responsible. Similarly, none doubted that most women with implants were getting along fine.

The stories doctors presented as those their patients told them parallel the stories we heard directly from the women with implants we interviewed, but they varied according to the specialty of the physician. Rheumatologists told us of women with problems while we heard of the benefits to patients from plastic surgeons, the family physician, and gynecologists. We explore specialty differences in a later section.

Psychological Causes

The controversy over silicone gel implants has turned to whether silicone implants have led to patients' problems; one alternative explanation says that the problems are psychological rather than the result of implants. The doctor in our very first interview began by telling about the only patient who had told him of any difficulties with her implants:

> My first experience with an individual patient is one who came to me with a story that the silicone had spread to her uterus and ovaries and has caused her now to have irregular periods and was really borderline as far as her personality. I'm sure there is neurosis, if not a psychosis, there of some sort. But a woman who'd had implants obviously read about what the possible scenario might be with the consequences. . . . Within 48 hours of seeing me and my reassuring her that there was no evidence that there was any relationship to uterine or ovarian problems (I could certainly come up with far better explanations of her menstrual disorder) she was interviewed on one of the local television stations. . . . She's the only patient that has come to see me with a gynecological complaint related to her silicone implants and she is convinced that it has traveled throughout her body and is responsible for any malady that might possibly occur.

This doctor went on to say that women who seek implants are different from other women. They are more concerned about their bodies and, hence, more likely to be aware of symptoms. If they experience the normal aches and pains of life, they are more likely to attribute them to something in the news like silicone gel implants.

The story troubled us. It might well be accurate. Certainly psychological issues would be important in a procedure undertaken because patients believed their appearance to others was worth expensive surgery, but this was also a women's health issue. We were wary of anything suggesting a sexist response blaming symptoms on women's "hysterical natures." A female psychiatrist friend had told us in casual conversation that she thought most women who sought implants had psychological problems. We pursued the question in subsequent interviews. When asked if implant patients were different from others, another gynecologist replied:

> Actually, probably when you think about it they are, but I don't consider most of them obsessive about it. They do, as a rule, have better body habitus. They fix themselves up more; they're more likely to wear makeup. But there is still a large fraction of people, a large group, that dress and appear just the same and have not had it [implantation].

His response is characteristic of most of the doctors we interviewed. There is a consensus that those who want implants, particularly those who seek them for cosmetic augmentation rather than postmastectomy reconstruction, are more aware of their appearance than are other women, but that awareness is not seen as extreme enough to be pathological or a likely explanation for their experiencing symptoms. Many women who do not choose to have implants have similar qualities. A family physician answered that she could not pick women with implants out from a group of women generally.

Interestingly, two plastic surgeons and a general surgeon view women who have had subcutaneous mastectomies as different from other women. One plastic surgeon talked about the amount of anxiety and fear of cancer that these patients experience before deciding to have a mastectomy because they believe that their fibrocystic disease will lead to cancer, due to a family history of breast cancer, or because of chest pain. Both this plastic surgeon and the general surgeon have stopped doing subcutaneous mastectomies. They argue that fibrocystic disease does not lead to cancer. Further, they are concerned that women who have the procedure in the hope of relieving breast pain are likely to be disappointed. Here they are joined by another plastic surgeon who believes these patients have unrealistic expectations that are not generally realized. The general surgeon explained that much breast pain is costochondritis (related to rib and cartilage). Forty percent of all his patients have such pain. If the pain comes from costochondritis, neither subcutaneous mastectomies nor implant removal will alleviate it.

One of the plastic surgeons felt so strongly on the issue that he regarded subcutaneous mastectomy patients as a group different from those who seek postmastectomy reconstruction or cosmetic augmentation:

> The most difficult to handle and deal with have been the women that have had subcutaneous mastectomies and breast reconstructions. . . . They, in general, have been the women with the most bizarre complaints. In a lot of women, if you go back through their history and say, "Why did you have the subcutaneous mastectomy to begin with?" A fair amount of women will say, "Well, I had pains. I had pains in my breasts. I had pains in my chest and I was in pain all the time. That's why I had the surgery done—to get rid of the pain." And afterward, they find, very frequently, that the surgery has not gotten rid of the pain.

Some doctors feel that women with subcutaneous mastectomies are more likely to relate symptoms to their implants than are women who chose implants for other reasons. If these women are also different in the emotional nature of their experiences and in unfulfilled expectations from the procedure and the implants, they may account for an important proportion of the reported problem. Their experiences might be reported in a more emotionally charged fashion, contributing to the perception by some physicians that some of the problems reported by patients are psychologically based.

Doctor–Patient Communication

Communication difficulties compound all kinds of human problems. Such problems appear to contribute to the difficulties experienced by some implant patients.

Patients who have experienced symptoms they regard as attributable to their implants gave us examples of problems communicating with some of their physicians (see chap. 2). Similar stories were repeated by their rheumatologists. The rheumatologists told what they remembered of narratives their patients had told them. A predominant theme was an unwillingness of doctors to talk sympathetically, or even talk at all, to patients who reported difficulty with their implants:

> Dave: Some women have said that . . . the plastic surgeons didn't want to talk to them. Have you heard that?

> Rheumatologist: Yes, that's true, yes, over and over again. You know part of their frustration is that they've not had anybody who has taken them seriously. The plastic surgeons have from the beginning told them that they were crazy or it's not from their implants or, "Go see a psychiatrist." The internist whose propensity is to be sympathetic feels like it's just something he doesn't know anything about and he can't make any reasonable attempt to help these people.

Another doctor reported stories from women who felt that plastic surgeons had dismissed their concerns about possible links between illness and implants:

> I have had some patients . . . who have said that when they called their doctor, who put their implants in, with this question that they had these symptoms and they were related to the implants, the doctors were rude to them and said they were going through menopause, or some other problem, or patted them on the back and said, "Don't worry, honey." That made them very angry.

Another told us:

> I have heard from my patients that they were turned down over the phone as soon as they mentioned they had implants and they were not feeling well. . . . I've heard stories about very unpleasant encounters. . . . The doctor just turning his back on the patients and just leaving the room.

In contrast, several plastic surgeons told us they made it a point to talk with their patients once the media began to publicize the stories of women who felt their implants were making them sick. One talked to any patient who called in and explained what he believed to be the facts. He offered to remove the implants at no charge if they wanted him to do so. Only one of his hundreds of patients felt that she was having some symptoms that might be connected to her implants, and he removed them for her. That doctor has sent written updates to his patients.

Another plastic surgeon wrote to more than 200 of his patients whose addresses he could locate and offered to talk with them and to remove their implants for no fee. Again, only one of his patients asked for removal. He said:

Plastic surgeons, when this first started, should have immediately contacted all their patients and said, "Gosh, there's this controversy and I really don't know what the answer is, but I want you to know that I'm very concerned about your health and I want you to come in and talk with me about that. I'm going to keep you up-to-date on everything that we know. If there seems to be any problem whatsoever, I'm going to take your implants out and I'm not going to charge you." If we had done that, we would have as our allies a million women with breast implants.

The relational impact of the communication pattern recommended by these two plastic surgeons seems clear. In the midst of uncertainty and anxiety, a strong, clear message of concern for the patient's well being was reassuring. It also opened the door for the possibility of an alliance with the patient.

In the interviews reported in chapter 4, women who did not feel their implants had made them ill reported much more positive interactions with their doctors than did women who attributed symptoms to their implants. The former liked and trusted their plastic surgeons. Some had selected their doctors because of past relationships, or judgments that the doctors communicated well. They felt that the communication had been helpful and that their doctors had talked to them as they had hoped they would.

The pattern described in chapter 3, in which physicians appeared to be unsympathetic and unwilling to listen to their patients, was associated with the opposite effect. Patients who thought they had problems felt rejected and sought others to help them. They told us and they told other doctors about that rejection. We do not have direct evidence that the communication patterns exacerbated their symptoms, but if being reassured and cared for often makes patients feel better, the opposite feelings are likely to make them worse. When these women found their doctors to be unsympathetic, they eventually turned to media accounts and to groups of other women as sources of diagnostic and treatment information. These sources reinforced the patients' alienation from doctors. Could better communication with their doctors have prevented their mistrust of medicine? Did the communication fail because the doctors were unable to provide acceptable diagnoses and symptom relief, or did poor communication contribute to diagnostic and treatment failures?

Cycles of trust contribute to the full expression of information and uncertainty on the part of both parties within relationships. Trusting relationships stem from and foster mutual liking. When doctor and patient like each other, they are more likely to accept difficulties as problems to be solved and work on them together. These cycles are likely to be self-reinforcing.

In just the opposite fashion, cycles of distrust can accelerate the deterioration of the exchange needed for good diagnosis, effective treatment, and patient willingness to implement treatments prescribed. As such relationships unfold, physicians and patients are less likely to be forthcoming with needed information or questions. They are likely to limit their time together. Dissatisfaction and mistrust will compound in the same self-reinforcing manner as trust.

But what initially determines the direction of the cycle? Before ascribing blame to either physicians or patients, we should note that we have no direct observations of what really happened in the doctor–patient communication. We are reporting thirdhand, secondhand accounts of experiences remembered by patients who have been unhappy with the medical outcomes. It is plausible that patient memories of what happened were interpreted in light of their subsequent unhappiness.

Yet, some of the doctors we talked to also felt that their communication with complaining women was problematic. After all, the large majority of their patients did not express such difficulties. They described the complaining patients as difficult to talk with:

> When I hear women saying on TV and in the newspaper that plastic surgeons won't remove their prostheses, I can only think of one who came in and I asked her what she wanted to do. . . . She didn't have a real problem, and she told me—or at least I thought she told me—that she wanted to keep them. And I said, "Well that's fine. Let's see you again in about 3 months . . . let's send you to see Dr. So and So to get the mammogram repeated that you want and come back and see me in 3 months." About a month later, she called and was the angriest woman I've ever seen . . . She'd been to see another plastic surgeon who had told her she needed her prostheses taken out. . . . [She asked] why couldn't I understand that?

There was general agreement that those with breast implants who had experienced rheumatological symptoms were difficult patients; patients with lots of questions, patients who took up a lot of the physician's time. One rheumatologist stopped seeing these patients entirely, in part, because of the time it took to talk with them thoroughly. Two other rheumatologists limited the number to four implant patients each week. The general surgeon who sees women about implant removal limited the number of these new patients to two weekly. One doctor told us:

> It's just a tremendous undertaking to try to sort them out. You really need a couple of hours with each patient. . . . And they are also very difficult patients. I mean, you are talking about people who come in with stacks of records. You're talking about interaction with lawyers. . . . And some of these people are very demanding. They sort of want everything done today or tomorrow. They're on the phone to find out results of laboratory tests a day after they are taken.

A rheumatologist explained:

> These are very meticulous persons. . . . Many are perfectionists, and, probably, that's what led them to get cosmetic surgery . . . and some have had more than one cosmetic surgery. . . . Most of them really have so many things to say that it takes easily 1 hour to see a new patient. . . . You have to try to filter the information and try to maintain the interview within a reasonable time frame and try to control the interview because, otherwise, the patients will keep going and going for more than an hour. That is different from what you see in the average patient that . . . comes in with a very defined set of symptoms and conveys information to you. But these patients, many times, can get diluted into many, I mean hundreds of, symptoms.

Another doctor told about running out of ink because the patient had so many symptoms to describe to him. Others spoke of long lists of complaints brought in by patients, some that appeared to be on printed forms rather than personally handwritten. You might recall from chapter 2 the 20 sick women we interviewed reported 80 different symptoms among them. How are doctors likely to have responded to such long lists, some that appeared to have been prepared by someone other than the patient?

The sheer length of the symptom list is likely to have led some doctors to reject the likelihood of a somatically based complaint in favor of a psychosomatic one. Doctors use the presence and absence of particular symptoms that differentiate and make diagnosis possible. When the patient seems to have everything wrong, symptom after symptom, then differentiation seems impossible. Perhaps the cause is not a specific illness, the doctor might conclude, but a problem in the patient's perceptions. If the patient copied somebody else's symptom list, perhaps in a support group, or had a diagnosis suggested by a television program or newspaper story, the doctor may be even more likely to attribute the illness experience to the patient's suggestibility.

Ironically, the fact that the sick women had so many symptoms may have led some doctors to discount the symptoms in favor of the more general diagnosis of psychological difficulty. As the doctor's comments revealed this impression, the patient seems likely to have felt misunderstood, not listened to, and not taken seriously. Some of the complaints about physician communication we heard directly from patients, and from some of their doctors, may have derived from the multisymptom nature of their own stories.

We do not know how often implant patients and physicians had difficulty talking to each other. The women who are angry with their doctors are outspoken. They have told other doctors and the press about their frustration. Those who are happy with their doctors have had less reason to speak out. The physicians who told us about proactive efforts to communicate with their patients report better experiences. But it may be that communication difficulty increases when problems are complex and unusual. The women who have had the most physical problems they connect to their implants seem also to have found greater difficulty achieving effective relationships with physicians, for whatever reason.

IMPLANT EFFICACY

As a result of the controversy over its use in breast implants, silicone has become a suspect material. It has been indicted, if not convicted, of causing illness. Silicone gel has been the most frequently used material for breast implants. It had been thought to be a safe and highly efficacious material by the plastic surgery community. It was believed to be inert; nonreactive in the human body.

One plastic surgeon talked about the progress that silicone implants represented:

We had worked a long time to find a material that was acceptable. I came through an era when we used the Ivalon sponge . . . and some other things. One time, early in the game, there had been paraffin and other materials. And so silicone, to us, was a godsend, you know. It was a wonderful thing to have something that was not reactive.

Silicone is widely used in medical devices, finding its way into shunts, valves, coatings for pacemakers, lubricants for syringes, and other materials. It has been regarded as the best foreign material to put inside the human body.

Almost all the physicians interviewed agreed that silicone gel breast implants bring the desired results to patients. They referred to the findings of Iverson's survey (1991), that showed more than 90% of implant patients were satisfied with the devices.

The gynecologists we interviewed said they usually learned about patients' implants during a routine history or breast examination. All three stressed that their patients were overwhelmingly satisfied with their implants. One said, "As a rule, most of them that have had them done, I found, are very happy with the outcome. They think more of themselves, and it's a rare person who's unhappy after it's over."

Even rheumatologists, who believe that some women become sick because of an immune response to the silicone, reported that their patients were often reluctant to have their implants removed. Patients liked the difference in appearance that the implants have made and preferred not to lose that benefit. Implants were described as beneficial. They helped women who desired them. They are efficacious. All the doctors we talked to agreed that implants do what they claim to do. But do they do so safely? That is where the difference in views is most intense.

IMPLANT SAFETY

Implants and Cancer

On some issues, there is agreement between specialists. There seems little worry about a relationship between implants and cancer. Even before publication of the Alberta study, showing no statistical relationship between implants and breast cancer (Berkel, Birdsell, & Jenkins, 1992), there was little serious worry about implants increasing the chances of cancer. None of the doctors interviewed expressed that concern. There has been some belief that mammography might be less effective for women with implants, but the radiologists who read mammograms have felt that mammography could still be satisfactory (Ecklund, 1991; Fisher, 1992). Several of the physicians we interviewed expressed some reservations about the impact of implants on the success of mammography, but they did not suggest that as a reason for avoiding implants; only for care in getting and performing mammograms.

Side Effects, Contracture, and Rupture

Plastic surgeons did acknowledge some possible problems with the implant procedure. Plastic surgery is surgery. There can, of course, be side effects from any surgery. Although these are very real problems to the women who experience them, no one saw them as especially frequent following implants. Side effects such as infection seemed to be most frequently mentioned in our interviews in relation to the tram-flap operation, a reconstruction procedure using tissue and muscle from the patient's own abdomen to rebuild the breast. This more extensive surgery is a substitute for reconstruction using implants.

Despite early claims about the strength of the implants that suggested they could be run over by a car and not break, there was agreement that some implants do rupture. Opinion varied on how likely that is. In Iverson's (1991) survey, 6% of augmentation and 12% of reconstruction patients reported complications such as infection or rupture. Rheumatologists we interviewed seemed to believe the frequency was much higher. All subspecialists agreed that some small amount of silicone will "bleed" through the wall of the implant. The amount and impact of such bleeding, however, was a matter for considerable disagreement.

In addition, some women form very firm capsular contractures around their implants. The percentage of women thought to experience capsular contraction, hardened breasts, varied widely. Estimates were as high as 50% to less than 10% of patients. Capsular contracture is treatable through surgery. Some plastic surgeons say it can be prevented through massage. Although no longer recommended, many women underwent a procedure involving hard, quick, squeezing of the affected breasts. We heard of women whose breasts had become hard who were willing to undergo this often painful process more than once to keep their breasts soft.

The story we were told about the discovery of the squeezing procedure is interesting. A young woman had experienced capsular contraction and was to have surgery the next morning. She went to a party where a professional football player gave her an especially hard and painful hug. When she touched her breasts, which had hurt during the hug, she found them soft. The next day her plastic surgeon confirmed that the contracture had been broken down. A new treatment was born.

Many women with ruptures and contractures were satisfied enough with their implants that they had them replaced rather than removed. We heard of women who had several such replacements. Some reported having as many as eight sets of implants.

Connective Tissue Disease

A matter of major interest has been the claim that the silicone gel in implants can be related to rheumatological disorders sometimes called human adjuvant disease, sometimes called silicone associated connective tissue disease, and sometimes referred to as autoimmune disorders. Here, the views of physicians differed markedly. Some rheumatologists, initially only a small number, believed that they have seen cases where patients' rheumatological symptoms can be attributed to the silicone from their implants.

The rheumatologists, who believed that silicone is related to symptoms they saw in women with implants, told us that silicone gel can enter the body from the rupturing of the implant shells and that even the shells themselves can "shed" microscopic silicone particles. In women sensitive to silicone, this small amount can be sufficient to cause symptoms. One described a case early in his experience:

@EXTRACT = We were both seeing patients that had breast implants and rheumatic disease signs and symptoms, but the assumption was that this is a coincidence. So, the first patient that sort of impressed me beyond that was a lady who came in with a pain in her upper back and neck, and about in 1984 she was working in a fan store and lifting some boxes and, you know, it wasn't clear what was going on. I considered fibromyalgia. I also considered polymyalgia. I gave her a week of cortisone to see if it made any difference and it didn't. . . . We treated her with darvocet and tricyclics and she didn't, you know, get much better. It just sort of persisted. I don't believe I even knew she had breast implants at that point. I don't recall, but I saw her once every 6 months to once a year for a couple of years. And about 1986 she sought me out in the hall and said, "Listen my breast implants eroded through the skin and I took them out and I'm feeling so much better. You know, my muscle pain in my upper back and neck is gone."

Surely, if the patient improved once her implants had come out, there was reason to consider a connection between implants and the cause of her symptoms. The doctor went on to describe a patient with very severe symptoms resembling lupus who had been referred to a colleague:

> The lady looked like she was going to die so he gave her 30 of prednisone. . . . They took out her implants and [she] got dramatically better. In fact, she went from looking like she was going to die to being pretty much a normal person. In fact, the last time I saw her, now 4 years later, she was back at work at McDonald's, 11 hours a day, having a few aches and pains, but . . . for somebody 55 or 60 who's working 11 hours a day at McDonald's, I thought it was pretty good.

To continue to pursue the connection, a research fellow was assigned to collect the case information on patients with breast implants who had rheumatic symptoms, and had had the implants taken out. Of 11 cases identified, 10 were doing better after the implant removal. These cases were reported at the national rheumatology meetings in 1989.

Another rheumatologist explained his experiences differently. He began to review the literature on silicone for an academic lecture:

I really was amazed at all the literature on this. Certainly all the human data is anecdotal, but there really is a lot of material, and a lot of it, early in particular, came from plastic surgeons . . . there is also a reasonable amount of laboratory data at least putting silicone in laboratory animals and seeing the results. So it became obvious to me on reviewing the literature that there really was a lot of work and all of it pointed to the fact that silicone was not biologically inert.

If silicone is not inert, then people could react to it and have symptoms that might bring them to a rheumatologist. He agreed to see patients:

And my experience with seeing those patients is that, while this is totally anecdotal, there are . . . certainly women who react biologically to silicone and develop a clinical problem. Now, I don't know what the numerator is on that. I don't know how many women develop a problem, but with . . . the tremendous number of women who want to come here to be evaluated from across the country, it doesn't seem to be a small number.

Ironically, the number became so great that he felt the rest of his practice had been overwhelmed and he decided to discontinue seeing these women as patients.

The view of most plastic surgeons early in the controversy was that there was no scientific evidence linking silicone gel implants and rheumatological disease. Further, they argued that millions of women had received these implants over many years. Surely, they say, if there was a problem, plastic surgeons would have noticed it. The plastic surgeon who had served on the FDA panel said:

Every legitimate scientific organization in the country and in the world . . . came to no other conclusion than that the data indicated silicone gel implants were safe. . . . Most of the major rheumatological associations and major centers . . . have failed to identify any association of silicone gel implants with any known immune disease.

Another plastic surgeon gave the interviewer a copy of the statement released by the American College of Rheumatology on February 12, 1992, which quotes the FDA Advisory Panel as saying, "There is no convincing evidence that these implants cause any generalized disease. . . . the likelihood that any symptoms are related to silicone implants is extremely low" (Sergent, 1992).

Plastic surgeons consistently referred to the evidence presented by the rheumatologists as merely anecdotal, not scientific. One called it "junk science." Another said:

The opinion of the American College of Rheumatology [is] that there's no link between any of these rheumatological problems or autoimmune problems and breast implants. The FDA says the same thing. The American Society of Plastic and Reconstructive Surgery says the same thing. There's no convincing medical evidence linking silicone gel with autoimmune disease.

Not all plastic surgeons or rheumatologists agree completely with their colleagues. The rheumatologist on the FDA panel was the author of the statement by the American College of Rheumatology. Indeed, the problems with silicone gel implants have not been featured prominently in the rheumatology literature. Among the plastic surgeons interviewed, there was some acknowledgment that there might be a problem with silicone for a very few women. Even the Society of Plastic and Reconstructive Surgery modified its position, somewhat, by establishing a fund to underwrite research on the issue. The three gynecologists and the family physician we interviewed accepted the FDA position that only women with symptoms should worry about their implants. Three of the four had not seen a patient who had implants and symptoms. The fourth had seen one patient with menstrual problems whom he believed to have much more likely causes for her problems than her implants. Because these physicians had seen substantial numbers of patients with implants and none with problems, they, quite reasonably, believed any connection to be rare, if present at all.

Different specialists held different opinions about the safety of silicone gel implants. The rheumatologists we interviewed had seen cases that convinced them that implants were potentially harmful at least to some women. The plastic surgeons repeatedly referred to the absence of scientific data showing a danger. The family physician and gynecologists had not seen patients with problems and were inclined to discount the claims of danger. How can doctors looking at patients, sometimes the same patients, and reading the same literature come to such different conclusions? The physicians' perspectives on the relationship between science and knowledge proved helpful as we tried to understand the doctors' diverse conclusions.

Good Science

If people of good conscience disagree on what the available evidence shows, it seems reasonable to ask what they think constitutes good scientific evidence. What would be required to settle the issue to the satisfaction of the various groups of physicians involved? One of the questions we asked of each physician was, "What would constitute good science that would give a definitive answer?"

There was less difference of opinion than might be expected. Almost all the physicians advocated long-term studies comparing women who had implants to those who did not. A rheumatologist said, "They should have taken the first thousand women who got them and a thousand of their best friends and checked on them every year for 20 years." A plastic surgeon argued: "The next step is to do hypothesis-based research, with the hypothesis that silicone gel implants that are leaking, resulting in silicone associated connective tissue disease. The null hypothesis is that they don't. You gotta' look at both groups."

A gynecologist called for "case-controlled, population-wide, epidemiologic studies":

The only good epidemiologic studies, in that respect, are very large and very broad both in terms of numbers of people and in duration. I think about menopausal estrogen in the cardiovascular disease story. We have been talking about it for 20 years, and only now have we had 30 years worth of data to be able to show a direct relationship. Yet, we can't take any individual woman and give her estrogen and prove that it cuts her risk for heart disease in half. But we can take three million women over a 20-year period of time and look at the incidence of takers and nontakers. I think that's good science.

Several other physicians looked toward the discovery of evidence of "a body substance or a secondary immune function or something that would show that these patients with implants have something in their systems that patients without implants don't have," or an antibody to silicone. One said, "If they're postulating that a microgram amount of silicone is going to be enough to induce an autoimmune reaction, then it must be an incredibly strong antigen and there should be huge amounts of women who are having the problem." It follows for him, then, that a large national study would be a good test. One interviewee hoped for discovery of a genetic marker. Overall, they agreed on what a definitive scientific effort should involve; a large-scale epidemiologic study over a number of years accompanied by laboratory work to discover whether an antigen can be found.

Implant Removal

One further test of scientific knowledge might be found in the results of implant removal. Because a number of patients diagnosed by the rheumatologists have had their implants removed, it ought to be possible to learn something by observing what happens to their health after removal. But there was some disagreement. One plastic surgeon studied the outcomes:

Of the first 30 or so we looked at, we broke them down into two groups. . . . Those patients who met all the criteria of the American Rheumatological Association for diagnosis of connective tissue disease and . . . their symptoms did not improve after implant removal. This other group was composed of women who didn't meet the criteria for diagnosis of connective tissue disease, but they had symptoms, joint pain, muscle pain, fatigue, and they may or may not have had abnormal laboratory studies. . . . Probably 60% percent say they're better; 40% percent are unchanged.

The rheumatologists, on the other hand, believed that most of their patients have done better following implant removal. The specialist disagreed about the medical outcome of implant removal even though most of the patients studied by the plastic surgeon came from the rheumatologists' patients. The rheumatologists wanted a longer follow-up time than the plastic surgeon's study had used. The two specialties also used different measures. The rheumatologists relied on clinical observation, whereas the plastic surgeon used patient self-reports. One of the rheumatologists felt that the data should be taken more seriously because it approached the statistical region of rejection.

When the general surgeon was asked whether patients did better after removal, he replied:

> Yes. Yes. But I also tell patients that a clear 37% of patients will have a placebo effect. And I tell this to the patient. If I were to bring you in here and tell you that, "if I made an incision here, it would cure you of your problem," 37% of the patients who had an incision here would be cured of their symptomatic problem.... You would expect at least 40% of your patients initially to have a positive outcome from the removal of the implants even if there was absolutely no relationship.

Another plastic surgeon told of a patient he did not believe had an implant-related problem who had been so diagnosed by a rheumatologist. She insisted she wanted her implants removed so he agreed to do it. He gave her a local anesthetic, which meant she was awake and aware during their removal. As soon as the first implant was removed, before the second was out, she declared that she was cured. Her symptoms were gone. The plastic surgeon, believing that no real somatically based illness could be cured so quickly, took this as evidence that her problems were psychological. Such patients would seem especially likely to improve on removal of their implants.

We cannot draw clear conclusions about the results of implant removal from our interviews. The method of determining outcomes was not agreed on, the time period in which improvement was to be noted was not standardized, the placebo effect was not controlled, and the role, if any, of psychosomatic symptoms was not clear.

A rheumatologist expressed what a number of doctors said, based on the removal of silicone gel implants from the augmentation market, "It may well be too late to do any science on this because you'd have to have a placebo controlled study. You'd have to have matched groups." All seemed to agree that the FDA's action restricting implants means that the studies will not be done. Few expected silicone gel implants to be back on the market.

DIFFERENCE BETWEEN SPECIALTIES

Clinical Knowledge

If there was much agreement about science, physicians expressed much disagreement about what to do with knowledge of clinical cases. All doctors rely on clinical experience to guide them in decisions about diagnosis and treatment. But can one argue for the existence of a disease process on the basis of clinical experience? Here the specialty differences between plastic surgery and rheumatology became relevant. Plastic surgeons literally see concrete problems, have clear procedures to follow, and can see how successful they have been. Rheumatologists, by contrast, work with vaguer symptoms and often help patients manage, rather than cure their illnesses. One rheumatologist described his specialty:

Rheumatology every day is an environment in which there is no definitive test for anything. An ANA doesn't make the diagnosis of lupus. Rheumatoid factor doesn't make the diagnosis of rheumatoid arthritis. Everything is based on clinical findings and what the history of the patient tells you and the physical exam. . . . We're not like infectious disease. We can't get a positive streptococcal culture from a throat and a hundred people in a row can agree, "That's strep throat." Rheumatology is filled with theoretical constructs. When illnesses don't quite fit what exists . . . on clinical grounds you can tell, if you're a good rheumatologist, that its a little bit different from the natural disease. So, that's why I'm satisfied that the syndrome exists. But again, my observations—I've never said they were the definitive scientific study . . . or even scientific at all. It depends on how you use the term. I consider myself a scientist and I consider my observations scientific in the sense that I'm making them carefully. But from the standpoint, is my data the scientific study everybody's been looking for? No.

The general surgeon described the absence of definitive tests in rheumatology and the high level of ambiguity in rheumatological practice:

If I were a rheumatologist, how would I think? I'm treating patients with no known cause of their diseases. Ninety percent of the disease processes I treat have no known cause, have no good treatment that's definitive, and are chronic in nature, and the patients continue to progress and do poorly over time. And so, finally here now there's a possible cause for a disease process that's so frustrating, as a physician, to treat and deal with. You know, certainly the gut reaction has got to be "I've now found an actual etiological cause for a problem that we've never to date been able to figure out the etiological mechanism of, and we've never been able to treat. We have a potential for treatment in at least removing these things and we've seen some positive results by doing so."

When rheumatologists describe these cases, however, plastic surgeons call them "mere anecdotal evidence." They regard the symptoms as vague, perhaps psychologically based. The symptom list is too long and it has too much variability for plastic surgeons to accept the diagnosis of a single disease.

It became apparent from our conversations that the differences in the way the two specialties practice medicine generates very different regard for cases as evidence. Plastic surgeons can look at the patient problem they must treat, have clear procedures for treatment, and can easily observe how successful they have been. Their clarity is the antithesis of the ambiguity in rheumatology. Plastic surgeons rely on their clinical experience to guide their skill in the performing of procedures, but when it comes to case description and diagnosis, they are not accustomed to dealing with the uncertainty that characterizes rheumatology. Surely some of their disagreement about the usefulness of case examples is founded on the difference in their daily practice.

Ironically, of course, the plastic surgeons we talked to offered case examples to try to illustrate instances in which the rheumatologists had been wrong about cases.

The examples are interesting in their own right. One plastic surgeon described patients who had been diagnosed by a rheumatologist as having silicone-based disease:

> I have had patients whose complaints, I think, were pretty amazing that anybody would say they were related to their implants. For instance, . . . they have pains that feel like lightening bolts shooting off the tops of their heads and they've been told that this is related to their implants, and if they have their implants removed the pains in their head will go away.

We heard three different versions of a story about a case presented by a rheumatologist at a plastic surgery professional society meeting. The patient was described as having axillary pain and a fibrous band running down her arm. The doctor showed a slide of the patient's arm and explained that the problem resolved within 2 weeks after the removal of her implants:

> So I show these pictures . . . and the plastic surgeons all yell "Mondor syndrome." Of course I have no idea what Mondor syndrome is. But later I go to the library and I find out that Mondor syndrome is thoracal epigastric thrombophlebitis. . . . Obviously that's not in the arm so it couldn't have been Mondor syndrome if you're going to be strict. But it wasn't even thrombophlebitis.

A plastic surgeon in attendance at the meeting tells the story differently:

> He brought with him a slide of a patient that had silicone disease as a reaction to a leaking prosthesis. He showed this and it was Mondor syndrome which is a thing I thought everybody knew about, a reaction of the soft tissue and vasculature. . . . This patient had the prosthesis removed and got better in a couple of weeks which is about the recovery time that you would expect. And he showed this and didn't even recognize a sophomore level clinical entity. . . . Everything he said was of that ilk of information. I was not impressed with his clinical acumen. He was certainly unscientific in his views. . . . I just didn't think his medical knowledge was of the level that it would require to accredit these views.

This doctor regarded the lack of knowledge of what he took to be common medical information to prove the lack of clinical and scientific competence on the part of the rheumatologist. If he does not know such an obvious fact, his other knowledge and judgments about cases become suspect as well. As a matter of curiosity, we asked four internists, several very prominent in academic circles, to explain Mondor syndrome. None had heard of it.

In one more example, a plastic surgeon told of a patient who arrived with her complete medical records. She had been diagnosed by a rheumatologist as having silicone disease. When the plastic surgeon went through her records with her, he was able to find each of her numerous symptoms diagnosed before she had the implants put in. Again, the judgment of the rheumatologists' clinical acumen was discounted.

Plastic surgeons and rheumatologists practice medicine differently, particularly in how they proceed in the face of uncertainty. They regarded case examples as playing different roles in medical knowledge. They differed in their reaction to the cases of a number of patients they saw in common. This difference about the usefulness of cases accounts for much of their difference in medical judgment.

Referral Bias

One additional explanation of the different conclusions based on clinical experience might be called *referral bias*. The gynecologists and family physician we talked to had not regarded the silicone gel implant problem as very serious because they had seen virtually no implant patients with symptoms. They had not been moved to study the issue in the professional literature. They admitted that most of their information had come from the newspapers and from material sent to them by plastic surgeons. Yet, these are the doctors women would be likely to consult for advice. Many women had done so during regular checkups, pap smears, or breast exams. Because these women were not sick, asking only for reassurance, information, and guidance, their doctors concluded, from the sample of patients they had seen, that silicone implants presented little or no difficulty.

Referral bias exists for both plastic surgeons and rheumatologists. The general surgeon spoke of this:

> That dichotomy exists between the rheumatologist and the plastic surgeon. Here's a guy who sees 99% of his patients doing well with implants. The point is that the perception of the problem is so different. Here's a group of surgeons, physicians, who feel there is no problem because they see it so rarely. Yet, the rheumatologist is seeing all the other end of the spectrum. They never see a normal. They never see an implant patient with no problems. They always see only the implant patient with problems.

Women who experienced the kind of symptoms the media reported would not ordinarily go to a plastic surgeon for help even if they had previously been cosmetic surgery patients. They would be likely to visit other specialists and, after a time, might see a rheumatologist.

It is not surprising that rheumatologists and plastic surgeons see this issue differently. They see different problems in their practices. Their clinical experience is dramatically different. Because the Tampa Bay area has become a place where women with implants will get a sympathetic hearing from rheumatologists, patients come from across the country and the referral bias intensifies.

The differences in the level of uncertainty in ordinary practice, in the view held of case-created knowledge, and in referral bias seemed to account for the difference in views of those physicians who believed that silicone implants were linked to disease, and those who did not think so.

CONCLUSION

What can we conclude from these conversations with physicians involved with the silicone gel implant controversy?

First, because so much of what was said by parties in the controversy questioned the professional competence and motivation of the physicians involved, we listened quite carefully to those we interviewed. None seemed to be villains. Despite the charges in chapter 3 that plastic surgeons are too interested in money to care about their patients' well-being, we found no indication in the words or nonverbal behavior of any of our plastic surgeon interviewees that indicated a lack of concern for patients, for giving good care, and for following the best medical information. Several told us that their incomes were down as a result of fewer patients seeking implants, but for none did that seem an important influence. They were concerned that accurate facts be known. They were willing to counsel concerned patients without charge. Several offered to remove implants free for those who so requested. There were frequent, subtle indications of caring about patients throughout all the interviews. They talked about patients in caring ways. They expressed concern about patient well-being. The plastic surgeons seemed chagrined about those cases where patients had misunderstood them or not done well.

Despite the public criticism of the rheumatology group for being too outspoken about a possible connection between silicone and illness, there was no indication of anything but thorough, careful attention to patient well-being by those rheumatologists. They do seem attentive to evidence. They regard their clinical case experience differently than do their critics. They believe they need to act early to protect patients even if all the scientific data is not yet in. Throughout, it was clear that they wanted to help their patients. None of the responses of any physicians could be explained as the result of professional incompetence, or a desire for personal profit exceeding the doctors' concern for patients.

Second, despite all the argument about implant safety, the scientific differences of opinion between specialists may not be all that great. The relationship of implants to cancer does not seem to be a major concern of any of the doctors we interviewed. In addition, the claims made about rheumatological symptoms caused by implants are less disparate than they first appear. The sharpness of the disagreement about the relationship between silicone gel implants and various rheumatological symptoms is surprising when the actual nature of the claims made is examined. Plastic surgeons said that there is not any convincing research evidence on large numbers of patients showing a greater presence of rheumatological disease among silicone gel implant patients. The rheumatologists agree. No such studies existed at the time of these interviews. The strongest claim that the rheumatologists made was that for a small percentage of women, something about silicone might cause problems. They did not claim to have definitive scientific knowledge, but they did claim to have considerable clinical case information that argues for attention to the problem. None of the plastic surgeons we talked to was willing to say that no patient could ever have symptoms related to her implants. They all agreed that for a small number of women in relation to the total numbers who have received implants, a problem was possible. They all agreed that no epidemiological study had established such a linkage, nor had the mechanism for an etiology been discovered in the laboratory.

If the two groups can focus on the modest nature of the claim, they might be able to begin to talk to each other effectively about means of generating data that could shed more light on the issue. If antibodies or genetic markers indicating sensitivity to silicone are discovered, for example, patients likely to suffer symptoms could be identified prior to implantation. If more careful investigation of women whose symptoms are not related to silicone were undertaken, ways might be found to help them. They would not have to fall back on blaming silicone. All the physicians complained about the media and the FDA. Communication and cooperation within medicine could enable the two physician groups to influence the press and the regulators more positively.

Although doctors agreed on what would be good scientific evidence, they disagreed about what to do with clinical information about cases. Some emphasized cases as a guide to protecting patients from possible risks; others emphasized the sacrifice of possible benefit to patients in generalizing from an inadequate sample of cases not randomly selected. It would be interesting to invite both groups into a dialogue on the way clinical experience should inform medical practice.

Third, the efficacy of implants was not questioned by any doctors interviewed. Nearly all supplied evidence that implants have helped the women who have had them. Even doctors especially worried about implant safety told stories about patients benefiting from implants. Perception of benefit can balance perception of risk. It is the balancing process that is crucial in decisions about health risk.

The differences in physician perceptions between specialties can be partially explained by the differences in the way they practice and by referral bias. In looking at medical practice, generally it may be useful to see the differences in what doctors actually do. The rheumatologists and plastic surgeons proceed so differently, particularly in their response to uncertainty, that it is not surprising that they see the patients and outcomes differently. All doctors are not the same in the way they practice. Understanding those differences may enable us to understand and use doctors more effectively.

Fourth, doctors' perceptions of the difficulty in communicating with implant patients, particularly those who have decided that their implants have made them ill, balance, at least in part, the criticism of doctors by those patients in chapter 3. All the physicians agreed that these patients take more time and patience to talk with. Although we may not know who to blame for the communication failure, and assigning blame is usually not helpful in resolving misunderstanding, we do know that the conversation has been difficult from both perspectives. When patients have poor medical outcomes, doctors are likely to face obstacles in keeping relationships positive and productive. It would be interesting to assess what happens to doctor–patient communication generally when outcomes of treatment are poor. Even more useful would be a catalog of behaviors that seem to assist in maintaining cooperation in the face of such outcomes.

In an era where new scientific information has enabled so much improvement in medical care and health, we have become accustomed to expecting progress from new drugs and devices. Yet, much health information and medical knowledge is characterized by ambiguity, uncertainty, and contradiction. Risk is part of treatment. We are not yet very good at understanding that risk, and in dealing with the uncertainty. Despite the fact that they often talk about probabilities, physicians also have much to learn about how to deal with uncertainty. The silicone breast implant controversy stands out as an example, both because of the spotlight provided by the media and because of the dramatic way the actors have played their parts.

6

RATIONALITY AND NARRATIVE: MEDIA STORIES ABOUT SAFETY AND RISK

The story of breast implants isn't the simple one it once seemed—not a story of technology triumphant over the limits of the body, but one of wishful thinking, greed, and gullibility. The drama being played out now is equally complex, and there's no subtextual analysis available for the women who have unwittingly been assigned roles. (Davis, 1992, p. 170)

Magazine and newspaper headlines read: "Time Bombs in Breasts;" "The Implant Panic;" "My Breast Implant Disaster;" and the "Silicone Scare." Television anchors introduced stories with "Another health risk for women . . .;" "Another disturbing medical story . . .;" and referred to the "dangers of silicone implants." Between December 1990 and July 1992, the print and electronic news media told a public story about silicone breast implants: the women who had them, the plastic surgeons who inserted them, the companies who made them, the government agency that regulated them, and the scientific community that tested their safety.

These media accounts themselves comprise an important part of the implant controversy. We know that news media are significant sources of health information. Reviewing public opinion polls, Singer and Endreny (1993) concluded that "for certain classes of events, [including many illnesses] information about risk is likely to come neither from personal experience nor from any other interpersonal source but, rather, from the symbolic environment of the mass media" (p. 3). Studies such as Johnson and Meischke's (1993) analysis of breast cancer information concluded that "the public perceives the media to be the source of most of its health-related information" (p. 42). Other studies indicated that women are more likely to receive health information from friends, family, and the news media than from medical professionals (Kee, Teleford, Donaghy, & O'Doherty, 1993). Furthermore, magazines, newspapers, and television news provide not only information, but also influence attitudes and behaviors toward health risks (Singer & Endreny, 1993).

In the case of silicone breast implants, the news media appear to have played an especially powerful role. We know many women are receiving most, if not all, of their information about implants from the media. Our public opinion poll, discussed in chapter 9, indicated that at the height of the breast implant controversy, 94% of women got their breast implant information from television, 79% from newspapers, and 48% from magazines. Only 11% had received information from a health professional. As indicated in chapter 3, women who attributed illnesses to implants revealed a strong reliance on the news media for information, support networks, and even diagnosis. Women who were satisfied with their implants also attributed significant influence to the media, often blaming reporters for heightening fears unnecessarily.

The news stories themselves confirm that women saw the media as critical forums for health information. Many women featured in news reports indicated that their motives to "go public" with their implant story were to prevent other women from suffering what the storyteller had endured. Talk show host Jenny Jones encouraged other celebrities to come forward, "If they'll talk about it, we can start doing some good" (Jones, 1992, p. 62). In an article from the *St. Petersburg Times*, Janice Buck explained: "'How many women are going through what I'm going through?' . . . She 'went public' because 'I don't want other women to have to go through the search, when you know you're sick, you know you're dying, and no one can tell you what you're dying from'" (James, 1991, p. 10F). These women assumed that the media are powerful forums for health issues.

Clearly, newspapers, television, and magazines contributed significantly to what women knew about breast implants. However, interviews with doctors revealed a concern that the media overplayed the problems and sensationalized the issue, creating a negative evaluation of implants. Many doctors we interviewed claimed that, by relying on the media rather than medical experts for information, women experienced more fear and worry than was warranted by scientific studies.

Did the media create unnecessary fear? Did news stories create negative perceptions of implants? What does the media story of breast implants tell us? Although physicians argued that the media portrayed implants negatively, our initial analysis revealed that the news accounts presented both sides of the controversy. But, as we studied the media reports more carefully, we perceived major differences in rhetorical form between pro-implant information and anti-implant stories. We also found major differences in the proportion of harm and benefit attributed to the silicone implants. We believe these disparities created a compelling and persuasive case against breast implants.

COLLECTION OF MEDIA ACCOUNTS

We collected a variety of media accounts for analysis. Eventually, our collection included 64 newspaper articles, 55 magazine articles, and 60 national network television evening news segments. As we began the initial stages of our investigation, we collected relevant newspaper articles on the implants from the *St. Petersburg Times*. The *Times* has the largest circulation of the daily newspapers in the

Tampa area and is regarded, at least locally, as an outstanding newspaper. The largest share of its ownership is held by the Poynter Institute for Media Studies, an education and research center that strives to elevate journalistic standards. We found 47 articles printed in the *Times* during a 12-month period. This heavy coverage, nearly a story a week, reflects the intensity of interest in the issue in the Tampa Bay area. In addition, as we worked on our analysis and talked to acquaintances about our research, we received newspaper clippings from colleagues and friends who knew of our research. As a result, some reports from other newspapers found their way into our sample. Our newspaper collection eventually spanned the height of the controversy, from January 1991 through July 1992, including 64 articles.

Because magazines are often used by women as a source of health information (Johnson & Meischke, 1993), we also collected all breast-related articles from women's magazines that we found at several local newsstands between July 1991 and July 1992. Hoping to better understand the information that women might have received previous to the controversy, we also included magazine articles on implants from periodicals indexed in the *Reader's Guide to Periodicals* from 1960 to July 1992. Our magazine collection spanned 27 years, from the first popular article on breast injections in 1965 through July 1992.

When we completed the analysis of the public opinion survey described in chapter 9, it became clear that television news was the most prevalent source of implant-related information. As a result, we analyzed all news segments on breast implants that ran on the evening news on ABC, NBC, and CBS from December 1990 (the date of Connie Chung's *Face to Face,* which initiated the public controversy) through December 1992. December 1992 was the last date indexed as we began our television analysis. We obtained the news segments from the Vanderbilt Television News Archives.

PROCESS OF ANALYSIS

As we explored the media coverage of the implant controversy, we used a number of methods for analysis. We began with content analysis. Initially, intrigued by physicians' perceptions that the news was overwhelmingly negative, we simply looked for overt bias. If an article or television broadcast was constructed like an argument supporting a thesis against implants, we counted that essay as "negative." If the report was created as an argument with a thesis in support of implant safety, benefits, or availability, the account was labeled "positive." Letters to the editor and editorials were the most frequent cases of this type of report. If the article or news segment dedicated a majority of news space or time to a discussion of problems and/or support groups for women with implant problems, it was also counted as "negative." If the article dedicated a majority of news space to a discussion of benefits and/or support groups that promoted implants, it was labeled "positive." Articles and broadcasts with equal amounts of time or space dedicated to problems and benefits were coded "balanced or neutral." Also counted as balanced or neutral were articles and segments related to implants, but ones focused on topics that did not directly encourage a positive or negative attitude toward the implants themselves. Examples of this category included stories which described a change in leadership for Dow Corning or explained techniques for inserting implants.

This broad categorization of whole news accounts provided some support for the perception that news media were presenting a significant amount of bad news on breast implants. However, just as many news accounts balanced benefits with safety, the testimony of satisfied women with those who were ill, and accounts of efficacy with harm. Analysis of our news sample (see Table 6.1) revealed that 46% of the stories were negative, and 47% of the reports were balanced or neutral. Only 7% of the accounts were positive. Clearly the news of problems outweighed the reports of safety and benefits in those accounts that were overtly biased. However, most accounts were balanced or neutral. Missing were substantial numbers of reports devoted to implant benefits.

Wider differences appeared when the media were examined separately. Television news was considerably more negative than other channels. In total, 71% (43 stories) of television news segments were negative; and only 2% (one segment) had a pro-implant slant. In contrast, 42% (23 stories) of magazine articles were negative; and only 26% (17) of newspaper articles were negative. In addition, 63% (40) of newspaper articles and 51% (28) of magazine articles were neutral or balanced, and 16% (16 stories) of television news was balanced.

The analysis of overt bias provided us with a broad perception of the news coverage but we felt it was imprecise. We realized that our means of separating positive, negative, and balanced or neutral accounts missed more subtle and complex distinctions that emerged as we read the accounts. For example, articles that focused on manufacturers changing CEOs might not describe implants in a negative light, but nonetheless, might imply that the company was changing staff due to serious implant safety problems. In addition, a focus on whole segments missed the details within the news accounts.

TABLE 6.1
Overt Media Bias in News Accounts

	Number of Accounts	Negative	Positive	Balanced
Television	60	43 (71%)	1 (2%)	16 (27%)
Newspapers	64	17 (26%)	7 (11%)	40 (63%)
Magazine	55	23 (42%)	4 (7%)	28 (51%)
Total	179	83 (46%)	12 (7%)	84 (47%)

As we considered how the media accounts created impressions of breast implants and their safety, we found ourselves intrigued with the kinds of discourse that characterized different perceptions. We were interested in the fact that magazine and news stories presented a significant amount of good news for women with implants or women who were considering augmentation or reconstruction. Yet, it was the bad news that compelled our attention. Our survey, in chapter 9, showed that those who relied solely on media information sources were more negative about implants than those with nonmedia sources. Why?

One answer lies in the kind of discourse offered in support of pro-implant and anti-implant conclusions. Reports of implant safety and benefits relied primarily on abstract exposition, expert testimony, and statistics—the rational paradigm (Fisher, 1984). Reports of implant-related illnesses and problems relied more on dramatic narratives, often told in first person—the narrative paradigm (Fisher, 1984). The first person in the narrative paradigm accounts invited the audience to identify with the storyteller and provided a graphic depiction of the difficulties she experienced with her implants.

The news media frequently offered readers reassurance that implants were safe. News accounts included statistics and expert testimony that women have little to worry about and they often reported that the large majority of women were satisfied, "about 95 percent of the women who have had breast implants are extremely pleased with the results and have had no problems" (Landers, 1992, p. 7F); "less than one percent of women with implants appear to be having problems" (Mason, 1992, p. 3D); "one survey found that 71% of the recipients were 'very satisfied' with the results. Only 1% were very dissatisfied" (Kilpatrick, 1992, p. 16A). These statements were often repeated in the media. Yet, their rhetorical power was limited by the impersonal, abstract discourse of exposition, testimony, and statistics. In contrast, news about problems associated with implants were told in narratives detailing the struggles of women with implant problems.

A significant amount of coverage, particularly in the print media, was given to women with problems that are told in compelling narratives with full detail and human drama. These narratives often vilified doctors and implant manufacturers. A typical excerpt showing the contrast between narrative anti-implant material and abstract pro-implant exposition can be found in a *St. Petersburg Times* article:

"I think I've had a stroke," she told him over and over. She was 35 years old.

She was wheeled into the emergency room. "She's just having another anxiety attack," a doctor said. "I *told* you, you need to see a psychiatrist."

She had seen this doctor before, among many others in the previous two years, with one medical symptom after another: joint and muscle pain; burning in her pelvic area; bleeding ears; a mass (later found to be silicone) under her arm; scarring rashes on her neck; inability to concentrate. . . .

Doan says the effects are catastrophic. She cannot work, she is in pain, has unexpected attacks and difficulty concentrating. Her life is a question mark.

But even though Doan's experience is tragic, not unlike those of other women who have reported illnesses caused by silicone breast implants, there is no evidence that silicone is the culprit, many experts say. And surveys show the overwhelming majority of 2-million women with breast implants have had no problems and would recommend implants to others. (James, 1991, pp. 1F, 10F)

The stark contrast between the way the "good news" and the "bad news" was presented led us to use narrative analysis for greater understanding of the news articles describing the risk of implants. Analyzing the media discourse through the narrative analysis of plot, characterization, and setting enabled us "to evaluate the tale's rationality, the basis of its ability to influence belief and behavior" (Rybacki & Rybacki, 1991, p. 118). In our exploration, we traced major patterns in narrative structure: the content, the chain of events, and what happens to the characters in the tale. We asked how the plot identified problems to be solved, relationships to be worked out, and obstacles to be conquered. We looked at characterizations of major players and their relationships with one another. We examined characters' motives, their actions and the resulting consequences. In addition, we considered the contexts or settings in which the actions and plots unfolded.

Competing stories emerged from the discourse, but several narrative themes provide insight into the negative images that the media created about breast implants. The most compelling is the "horror story."

THE BREAST IMPLANT HORROR STORY

A primary focus of the media stories was on the woman who had implants and experienced major problems with them. These stories were comparable to the accounts told to us by women in chapters 2 and 3. Although the media sometimes reminded the reader that these women were few in number, "less than 1 percent of women with implants appear to be having problems" (James, 1991, p. 10F), much of the coverage featured detailed descriptions of their difficulties and trials, their motivations, and their unsatisfactory interaction with physicians.

These narratives detailing the struggles of women with implants were abundant and horrifying. The narrative structure that emerged from most accounts of patients with problems takes the form of a horror story in which the heroine acts to solve a problem (reconstruction following a mastectomy or low self-esteem caused by small breasts), encountering fearful challenges and difficulties along the way. The *St. Petersburg Times* explained the problems: "In the emerging controversy over silicone breast implants, this is a horror story. It is a worst-case scenario: A woman who may have a hypersensitivity to silicone receives a massive dose and suffers severe symptoms of mysterious origin. By the time the implants are removed, the silicone has migrated to other parts of her body" (James, 1991, p. 10F). Other media accounts reinforce the metaphor referring to specific, individual horror stories (Gould & Zucker, 1990, 1991a, 1991b) and a patient's "nightmare" (Sanders, 1992, p. 20). In these stories, the heroine begins confidently, trusting her plastic surgeon and his reassurances. Following the implant surgery, the woman experiences pain, mutilation, and unexplained illnesses. Trying to find relief, the heroine finds that people and events are not what they appear to be. Once-trusted physicians betray heroines by withholding support and critical information. The dream of a new figure fades in the realization of medical problems. Ultimately, fear and suspicion overcome faith. At the end of the horror story, the central character emerges sadder but wiser, often without her implants.

"Veronica's" story (a pseudonym) in *Ladies Home Journal* typifies the horror stories told in magazines, where the woman's narrative is elaborately detailed[1]:

In my mind, I equated breasts with womanhood itself: I believed that I was attractive, but I couldn't help feeling that somehow I wasn't a "real" female [because I was flatchested]. I also believed that a bigger bosom would be erotic and make me feel sexier. Yes, I wanted breasts. . . .

[After the surgery], I remember . . . waking up in the recovery room feeling an unfamiliar weight on my chest—two wonderfully perfect 36B breasts. . . . Late that night, I awoke in great pain. . . . My right breast was hemorrhaging, and the accumulation of blood had caused it to swell as large as a football. . . . [When that was fixed] my new figure made me feel liberated: I loved wearing bathing suits and backless dresses without worrying about a falsie slipping out of place.

Unfortunately, my euphoria was short-lived. Within a year, I began to notice that my right breast had hardened. . . . Worried, I went back to my surgeon, who told me that scar tissue had formed around the implant. He added that this complication was not unusual; however, this was the first *I* had heard of it. Still, I trusted my doctor. I needed yet another operation to remove the tissue. . . . Everything went well until about two years later, when I noticed . . . a small blister at the base of my right breast. . . . I went back to my plastic surgeon. . . . He confirmed my fear that the implant was being expelled, but couldn't explain why. . . .

In passing, the surgeon mentioned that the implant had a small hole in it. The leakage of gel had been minimal, he quickly added, so I had nothing to worry about. I took his word for it. . . . Several months [later] . . . my right breast still didn't look or feel right. Now I was livid; I'd had enough of this doctor and felt like a fool for having trusted him so long.

---

[1] © Copyright, 1992. Meredith Corporation. All rights reserved. Reprinted from LADIES' HOME JOURNAL magazine.

[After a corrective surgery by a second plastic surgeon] my implants continued to bother me. . . . My right breast began to harden again. I also noticed that when I leaned over or hugged someone I could feel my left implant sliding under the skin all the way to the top of my shoulder! . . . Not one of my doctors expressed any concern during my annual mammograms and exams. . . . I went to a third surgeon, who took one look at me and announced that I had a major rupture in my left implant. Since I'd waited so long to seek medical help, the implant might have been leaking for as long as five or ten years. Obviously these implants had to be removed, and the doctor recommend replacing them in the same operation. He insisted that the latest models were much less likely to harden or break. Besides I could always "pop them out". . . .

My initial impulse was to have the implants removed once and for all. Yet I wasn't sure I could face never having breasts again. . . . And the doctor made the procedure sound so easy; surely nothing could go wrong this time. . . . [During the surgery, the doctor discovered that] so much silicone had leaked out of the left implant that it was half empty! Furthermore, the right implant had also ruptured. . . . Thinking about what I'd endured for nearly two decades. . . . I listened to what my body had been trying to say from the start: Those implants did not belong in there. . . . [My doctor] argued that I would regret the decision, but my mind was made up. The surgery took an hour (so much for "popping them out"), and I awoke to find myself flat as a board once more. Yet I felt good: A burden had been lifted from my body and my life. (Sanders, 1992, pp. 20, 22, 24)

"Veronica's" story created a causal link between the implants and a series of detailed aesthetic and surgical complications. Such first person accounts provided a point of identification for the audience.

When televised, the accounts added graphic, visual confirmation. Janet Van Winkle's "8-year horror story" was told repeatedly in newspapers, magazines, and television, but nowhere more dramatically than on NBC's evening news on December 18, 1990. Describing the "horrible cost" that she paid for "big breasts," the news report showed pictures of how silicone migrated in her breasts, changing their shape from postimplant images of fullness to later pictures of odd breast placement and asymmetry. The pictures were so horrifying and explicit that NBC anchor, Tom Brokaw, warned viewers that the report included "graphic" pictures that viewers might find "disturbing" (Gould & Zucker, 1990). In a later magazine article, Van Winkel described the result, "My right breast was the size of a tangerine and my left breast the size of a grapefruit" (Eagan, 1992, p. 125). Pictures on television and in the magazine displayed oddly twisted breasts, scars, and disfigurement. The final photograph showed Van Winkel's mastectomy scars after her implants were surgically removed. While television flashed grotesque pictures of Van Winkel's mutilation, the reporter announced that she suffered from cancer and depression following her implants.

Just like Van Winkel, other heroines of horror stories faced disease as well as aesthetic complications. Kali Korn's story was told in the *New York Times* in 1991. Having undergone implant surgery "to enlarge small breasts, because she wanted to 'look sexy,'" Ms. Korn hoped to change her self-consciousness about her body:

As a teenager, Ms. Korn said, she was told she was "cute as a button" but flatchested. . . . She said she became very self-conscious about her body, "especially around men," who treated her like a delicate child. After getting the implants, Ms. Korn said, "somehow I felt sexy and men were different with me." Taped to her refrigerator are photographs taken after the implants and before she got sick. In the pictures, Ms. Korn's breasts spill from low-cut dresses. (Gross, 1991, pp. A1, A11)

Subsequently, ill from autoimmune disease, which her doctor blamed on her implants, Korn reported, "Now I could care less about men." The newspaper described Korn, "hobbling to the kitchen to show the photos." She is "forced to spend most of her time in bed." Blaming herself and her plastic surgeon, Ms. Korn remarked "I'm angry that I was told, 'Enjoy them,' rather than being told that somewhere down the line they might wreck my life. . . . I'm angry at myself for thinking implants would change my life and there wouldn't be a price." When Korn had her implants removed to relieve her symptoms, the surgeon found they had ruptured and the silicone had spread throughout her body (Gross, 1991, pp. A1, A11).

These horror stories create a repeated pattern of chronological sequences: healthy women have implants, then they suffer illness, pain, and/or mutilation. The women's narratives provide a chronological relationship between implants and illness. A causal link is implied.

The list of problems, which media accounts connected to implants, were many and varied. Most common were ruptures, leaks, autoimmune disease, hardening (capsular contraction), and cancer. The first four were often told dramatically in the women's accounts; they were usually described as severely painful. Media coverage of the cancer risk is explored in chapter 10.

The stories of ruptures and leakage were among the most frequent. Almost half of print news accounts included reports of implant leaks or ruptures. Some individual news stories made as many as eight references to ruptures or leaks (Eagan, 1992; Fischer, 1991). In Debra Doan's case, "240 cubic centimeters" of silicone escaped from her implant (James, 1991, p. 1F). CBS dedicated one news segment to the story of Sandy Richardson, a former television and film stuntwoman, who blamed her pain, fatigue, and memory failure on leaking silicone (Sorenson, 1991). Mariann Hopkins was the subject of many television, magazine, and newspaper accounts. Having won a 7.3 million dollar verdict against Dow Corning, "after her implants ruptured," Hopkins maintained that the silicone gel that spilled from her implants had damaged her immune system (Seligmann, Cowley, & Springen, 1992, p. 45).

In some accounts, such as "Veronica's" earlier horror story, the implants leaked outside the body. Cynthia Buford's decision to remove her implants came "after black goo began leaking from her nipples" (Rigdon, 1992, p. B1). Another woman called a patient hot line crying, "She noticed in the shower that her left breast felt squishy. When she looked down, she saw a greenish-beige gel leaking from her nipple" (James, 1992, p. 1D). A 33-year-old woman "found out that her implant had ruptured when a thin, jelly-like substance leaked from her right nipple and was identified as silicone" (Fischer, 1991, p. 98).

For "Veronica," Buford, and others, silicone migration—escape of the gel into other parts of a woman's body—was a common and graphic part of the story. Margaret Luker sought relief from pain "so acute just getting out bed was a 10-minute ordeal." When a surgeon removed her implants, he found that they had ruptured and had to recover "silicone that spilled even into her back" (Vick, 1991, p. 3A). Following a bilateral mastectomy, Barbara Johnson's surgeon assured her that her silicone implants would be intact for life. Two years later, her right implant ruptured. She replaced it and 4 years later she was told to expect lung cancer when a mass was discovered in her lung. Instead, further tests showed the mass was silicone that had ruptured and traveled to the lung (Eagan, 1992, p. 125). In a special report, *First for Women* magazine told the stories of celebrities who had breast implants. It included a picture of how silicone travels through the body, explaining, "Silicone is picked up and carried by the cells through the lymph system and into such organs as the spleen and lungs. . . . When a rupture occurs, large amounts may flatten out and move like a sheet of oil between the tissues" ("What price beauty?," 1992, p. 17). *Redbook* reported that "silicone from implants has been found in the spleen, thyroid gland, liver—even in the Fallopian tubes" (Fischer, 1991, p. 98).

Women's stories about leaks and ruptures were often followed by descriptions of autoimmune diseases, a series of symptoms "such as arthritis and lupus, in which the body attacks its own tissues. Those symptoms include fever, weakness, joint pain and skin rashes" (Seligmann & Church, 1992, p. 75). Autoimmune problems were the second most often reported implant-related side effect. They were cited in almost half of the print media accounts and one sixth of the television news segments. In a single article, the link between autoimmune disease and implants was raised 11 times (Fischer, 1991). Typical was a CBS news segment that explained the FDA voluntary moratorium on implants on January 6, 1992. The report focused on Sybil Goldrich, "one of several thousand women who claim they have health problems caused by silicone leaking from implants: cancer, diseases of the immune system, aching muscles and joints" (Sorensen, 1992a). *Mother Jones* reported that Janie Cruise's immune system declined following her implant surgery. Within days she experienced "severe pain in her left breast. . . . [the following year she experienced] severe headaches, fatigue, muscle and joint pain, numbness in her right hand, bronchitis, and gastrointestinal ailments" (Regush, 1992, p. 27). Anna Quindlen's syndicated column recounted Mariann Hopkins' experience, "She had spent years thinking that there was no link between her painful and debilitating connective tissue disease and the implants that she received after a mastectomy" (Quindlen, 1992, p. 8A).

Arthritis like pain was the most frequent autoimmune problem reported by women. Many women experienced crippling aches and immobility as a result of their implants: "Monteith walks with a slow and halting gait. She says she runs a continuous fever and wants only to get her health back. . . . 'Now my knees and legs are so swollen I can hardly walk'" (Ripley, 1992, p. 6B). Margaret Lusker described herself, "You know '*Old Man River*? . . . Body all achin'?' That was me" (Vick, 1991, p. 3A).

Scleroderma, an autoimmune disease resulting in painful hardening of the skin, was also represented in the women's accounts. Reports included charges by Stanley Drunker who said his wife was killed of scleroderma, "the skin becomes very tight, taunt, distorts the face, and results in pain" (Sorensen, 1992b). Kali Korn's autoimmune disease included scleroderma, the newspaper described her hands as "clawed, her skin . . . stretched as tight as plastic wrap, and she [could not] dress without help" (Gross, 1991, p. A1). Her doctor blamed the implants for her illness.

Implant hardening was the third most common individual complication mentioned in implant stories. About one third of the print media stories and one sixth of the television stories linked capsular contraction to silicone breast implants. Within a single story, breast hardening was cited as a problem as many as 12 times (Nashner & White, 1977). Jenny Jones' story featured in *People* magazine was the prototype example:

Eleven years ago this May, Jones underwent a breast-implant operation to increase her bust line and bolster her self-esteem. But like up to 15-20 percent of the estimated one million women in the U.S. who have implants, Jones ended up with lasting side effects. Her implants hardened, and vainly hoping to end her discomfort, she had them surgically replaced five times. (Jones, 1992, p. 57)

Jones' quest for relief included a series of unsatisfactory procedures and interactions with plastic surgeons who tried in vain to correct the problem. According to Jones, her original plastic surgeon underestimated the risk of capsular contraction. Six months after her initial surgery in 1981, Jones reported, "my breast got hard. . . . One insensitive male acquaintance told me when I hugged him goodbye, 'What do you have, rocks in there?' I was mortified" (Jones, 1992, p. 59). Her plastic surgeon replaced the implant free of charge, changing the size to see if that would make a difference. Jones explained, "It didn't. Within five months, my new implants started to get hard" (Jones, 1992, p. 59). Enduring a closed capsulatomy (where the plastic surgeon manually squeezes the implant to break up the scar tissue forming around the implant), Jones' implants hardened again. She underwent surgery a third time in 1983, to correct the capsular contraction, asking for a new kind of implant, the Même, that was not supposed to cause capsular contraction. Within a few months, the new implants were hardening as well. Unbeknownst to Jones, her plastic surgeon had replaced her earlier Vogue implants, not with the Mêmes, but with a replacement of her original type. When she had the Vogues replaced in 1984, her plastic surgeon finally did insert Même implants, which also hardened within months. Jones resigned herself to living with the problem:

I lived with them from 1984 until 1991. I resigned myself to the fact that my breasts weren't ever going to be soft. . . . Between 1985 and 1991, I went to one doctor after another—all men—asking, "Isn't there something you can do?" They all told me, "Be glad this is all that is wrong with you. Some women's breasts are as hard as cement." (Jones, 1992, p. 60-62)

In 1991, a different plastic surgeon told Jones that MISTI GOLD implants were available, which would make her breasts 50% softer. In March 1991, Jones underwent her sixth surgery and had her fifth set of implants. "In a couple of months, the MISTI GOLDS hardened too. My breasts were completely numb" (Jones, 1992, p. 62).

Jones' account was extreme. Few of the women who told their stories in media reports replaced their implants five times due to hardening, but many other women reported similar complications. Their degree of hardening varied from slight to intense. "Sue" got "new breasts" to attract men when she was 23 years old. Eight years later, "Sue's breasts have hardened somewhat despite the exercises she performed in the privacy of the company restroom" (Scheer, 1991c, p. A1). In contrast, other women reported augmented breasts that feel "like baseballs covered with skin" (Mithers, 1992, p. 84).

The women's stories of hardening, autoimmune diseases, ruptures and pain are compelling. These four complications are but the most frequently reported in the women's accounts. Seventy side effects or complications follow implant surgery in the personal narratives (see Table 6.2).

The number of complications that follow breast implants in women's narratives is impressive. The sheer repetition of these links compounded the impression of risk. Indeed, the vast majority of news accounts associated health problems, complications, dangers, and/or diseases with breast implants. Nine tenths of newspaper accounts, four fifths of magazine stories, and over half of television news programs mentioned at least one side effect or described risks linked to the medical devices.

TABLE 6.2
Health Problems Related to Implants in Media Accounts

Arthritis	Fibrosis	Nerve damage
Autoimmunne disease	Flu symptoms	Night sweats
Birth defects	Foreign body reaction	Numbness
Bleeding ears	Gangrene	Optical nerve damage
Blood blister	Granulomas	Pelvic burning
Botched surgery	Gynecological disorders	Pelvic pain
Breast discharge	Headaches	Poisoning
Breast pain	Heart attack	Rashes
Breathing problems	Human adjuvant disease	Reproduction problems
Bronchitis	Implant bleed	Rheumatological disorders
Cancer	Impaired circulation	Rib erosion
Capsular contraction	Infections	Ruptures
Chest pain	Inflammation	Scarring
Connective tissue disease	Insomnia	Scleroderma
Corrosion of implant	Joint pain	Silicone disease
Coughing	Leaking	Stiffness
Crippling	Lou Gehrig's disease	Stroke
Death	Lupus	Surgical complications
Depression	Mastectomy	Swelling joints
Discoloration	Memory loss	Swelling glands
Disorientation	Misshapen breasts	Swelling legs
Electric shocks	Muscle pain	Thyroid problems
Fever	Nausea	Traveling silicone
		Tumor

Most accounts listed multiple symptoms within a single article. For example, an early *Ms.* essay reported six different side effects in one article: "infections, deformities, excessive hardness, painful and disfiguring scars, emotional difficulties" (Nashner & White, 1977, p. 53). The essay also included several narratives that linked implants to multiple surgeries and hardening. Between the chronological links developed in the narrative accounts, the blame women attributed to the implants in the stories, and the repetition of associations in media exposition, the audience was left with a strong impression that implants lead to harm in a majority of cases.

The quest for larger breasts begins with high hopes and confidence. Along the way, women encounter illness, mutilation, and depression. What possible benefits could motivate women to take up such a journey?

BENEFITS

The news accounts frequently report on women's reasons. In *Reading the News*, Carey (1986) argued that media stories "explain actions by attributing motives. The motives they attribute are . . . rational, instrumental, purposeful ones" (p. 182). Within the news narratives, women act on clearly stated motives. Carey argued that such attributions can be arbitrary and may be described in such a way that makes the actors' purposes seem more clear than they really are. When the media reported the reasons that women had implants, the purposes emerged as trivial when compared to the risks and dangers.

The narratives presented two major motivations causing women to choose implants. They frequently mention reconstruction for breast cancer patients, "traumatized by the loss of a breast" (Craddock, 1992, p. 2B). Although reconstruction was mentioned about as often as the alternative motivation, breast enlargement, the motivation was rarely a part of any detailed narrative. Instead, reconstruction was usually mentioned as part of a statistical comparison between the numbers of women who seek implants for cosmetic purposes versus reconstructive purposes. The few fully developed stories in which women described the need for implants following mastectomies were printed before the public controversy over silicone implants began (Belson, 1983; Haupt, 1987; Seligman, 1980). As a result, it is the augmentation motive that dominated the news accounts during the period when the horror stories were presented. Breast enlargement was the motivation in most of the women's detailed narratives and was elaborated on in more detail.

As we looked at how the media treated women's augmentation motives, we were impressed by how minimal the benefits appeared. Trivialization occurred in four ways: (a) the juxtaposition of motives, (b) the use of minimizing adverbs, (c) the comparison of augmentation to cosmetics and fashion accessories, and (d) the commodification of implant surgery.

Magazines, newspapers, and television reports frequently compared statistics about motives indicating that most women chose breast implants to enlarge their breasts; far fewer chose the procedure following a mastectomy:

> The majority of women with implants sought them purely for the purpose of enlarging their breasts. But many got the implants as part of breast reconstruction after a mastectomy . . . and have praised the devices as important to their self confidence and sense of wholeness. ("Firm to Pay," 1992, p. 2A).

The comparison of augmentation to reconstruction as a motivation is implied in the choice of trivializing adverbs frequently attached to augmentation and enlargement motivations: Women receive breast implants "*just* to make their breasts bigger" ("Implants Likely," 1991, p. 3A; italics added), "*simply* to enlarge their breasts" (Craddock, 1992, p. 2B; italics added), and "*simply* to exaggerate their natural contours" (Cowley, Springen, & Hager, 1992, p. 56; italics added). The use of limiting adverbs like purely, just, and simply suggested that these motivations were not as noble or compelling as the reason a smaller number of women receive the implants: "restoring what has been lost" to cancer and to "not always be reminded that I had cancer" (Haupt, 1987, p. 78). Despite the fact that the comparison that trivialized augmentation motives included a broader and more positive motivation linked to cancer reconstruction, the media accounts during the implant controversy provided far more narratives about augmentation patients with detailed explanation of their motives.

Many accounts attributed augmentation to a cosmetic motivation, explaining that the "purely cosmetic" reasons were the most common ("Safety," 1991, p. 20A). Almost every article from the newspapers included a sentence similar to this one: "About 80 percent of U.S. women with breast implants got them for cosmetic reasons" ("Panel Advises," 1992, p. 1A). The stories often equated "cosmetic" plastic surgery with buying makeup or some other form of female ornamentation. One magazine reported that some doctors were using "newspaper ads that make nip-and-tuck look as easy as highlighting one's hair or coloring one's hair" (Regush, 1992, p. 26). Jennie explained that she got her implants as part of her fashion strategy to look better, "I felt it would look good. I love to look good. I dress well, I use a little makeup—it's just all part of it" (James, 1991, p. 10F). Implants were described by one woman as "fashion accessories" (Gross, 1991, p. A11). Another report referred to cosmetic surgeries as "aids to vanity" (Scheer, 1991a, p. A42).

Another trivializing theme presented implants as devices that helped women appear more attractive in their clothing. Many women reported using implants the way women previously have used girdles, padded bras, and fashion styles designed to camouflage figure faults. One woman got her implants 20 years ago in order "to look good in a bathing suit" when her husband put in a backyard swimming pool (Mason, 1992, p. 3D). Evidently her motive was shared by many. A *Los Angeles Times* series on plastic surgery explained that the demand for implants is "somewhat seasonal. A rise in the demand for breast implants coincides with the swimsuit season" (Scheer, 1991a, p. A42).

Complementing the swimsuit theme was a desire to look proportional. The *National Enquirer* reported that Dolly Parton had her "breasts enlarged in her mid-thirties, [when] she was gaining weight and felt her breasts weren't large enough in relation to her bigger size" (Capettini & Towle, 1992, pp. 1, 31). One plastic surgeon explained his patients' motives, "part of it is being able to fill out clothing" (Scheer, 1991a, p. A42). Comparing breast implants to makeup, a scarf, or a device for modifying one's figure trivializes the motive. Women often buy makeup, color their hair, and purchase fashion accessories for ornamentation, often at a whim.

The desire for breast enlargement was also trivialized by comparing the devices to the purchase of other consumer goods. Women do not undergo implant surgery, they "buy implants for cosmetic reasons" (Vick, 1991, p. 3A). The media reported women "purchasing breasts as a status symbol" (Scheer, 1991c, p. A10) and described the purchase not as a matter of health, but as a way to spend discretionary income. Plastic surgeon Malcolm Paul explained women's implant decisions as dependent on the economic cycle, "It's discretionary income. It's a new car, a family vacation, or a set of breast implants. It always follows that way, same as the car market, or the jewelry market" (Scheer, 1991c, p. A10). One woman, contemplating the operation, "view[ed] it as very much a matter of personal choice whether 'I forge ahead with a keen mind and a flat chest, or succumb to the pressures of society and buy a set of breasts like new silverware'" (Scheer, 1991c, p. A10).

Trivialized in comparison to breast reconstruction, women's motives for augmentation were "strictly" cosmetic. Compared to makeup or other fashion items, breast implants were often associated with the purchase of nonessential luxury items. The reader almost certainly inferred that such benefits, when compared to the problems associated with breast implants, were trivial. Some of the women's accounts made the judgment explicit, "It is not worth the price one must pay in the long run, sacrificing your health for the sake of vanity" (Mason, 1992, p. 1D). A reporter was just as direct in drawing public attention to the uneven comparison between benefits and harm: "Spending so much money on a potentially dangerous operation just to change the shape of some fatty tissue seems preposterous" (Mithers, 1992, p. 86).

Of course, not all motivations for choosing augmentation were minimized, but the more substantial reasons were presented as personal psychological problems that appear to be more appropriately solved by less risky and more therapeutic solutions. For women plagued by feelings of personal inadequacy, bad relationships, or obsessive concern over appearance, breast implants were described as a way to increase self-esteem and a sense of female identity. One augmentation patient recalls, "Marilyn Monroe and Brigitte Bardot were hailed as paragons of sex appeal, while at 16, I was tall and totally flat—my bony chest could have belonged to a young boy. . . . In my mind, I equated breasts with womanhood"

(Sanders, 1992, p. 20). Another chose implants because her marriage had failed and she needed a boost in self-esteem:

> Her seven-year marriage had just fallen apart, and she was facing re-entry into the singles scene. Encouraged by a close friend . . . Cruise handed over a few thousand dollars for what seemed like a miracle cure for her sagging self-confidence. (Regush, 1992, p. 27)

Following Timmie Jean Lindsey's augmentation surgery, she "found the self-confidence to seek out career guidance, counseling and a job that let her keep her family together" (Vick, 1991, p. 3A).

The need for increased self-confidence was linked, in many stories, to enduring feelings of personal and sexual inadequacy, "It grows out of years of feeling bad about themselves. . . . 'Before my surgery I knew I was a sexual being inside,' says Ambrose quietly. 'But when I was naked in bed, I just didn't feel right'" (Mithers, 1992, pp. 86, 90). Surgeon John Goin and Psychiatrist Marcia Goin explained the motivations of women they treated, "Women who seek augmentation often report having sexual difficulty. . . . Because these women are so self-conscious, they're unable to enjoy being fondled; some only feel comfortable having sex in the dark" (Mithers, 1992, pp. 88, 90).

Some media stories equated feelings of inadequacy with women's comparisons of their bodies to a socially constructed ideal. One reporter explained the problem:

> We develop the obsession. . . . we become increasingly convinced that only the perfect body is good enough. . . . If only we could slim down the fat places and pad out the flat places, we'd be sexy and desirable and beautiful and men would look at us and our husbands would love us and everything would be wonderful and we'd live happily ever after. Pathetic, isn't it? Intellectually, we know that. Yet we never quite believe that we can be feminine and sexy without big breasts. (Peters, 1992, p. 85)

Although improved sex lives and self-confidence seem like compelling benefits, the audience for the media stories was left with the impression that women should seek different solutions to these personal problems, especially given a perception that severe health risks accompanied the implant alternative. The ultimate lesson learned by women who sought self-esteem from implantation was self-acceptance, "My goal is to say to anybody who is considering implants: Don't do it. It's not worth the risk. Learn to love yourself. If I could have learned that, I wouldn't have had to suffer these 11 years of torture" (Jones, 1992, p. 62). The end of the horror story suggests that self-love, a shift in personal priorities, and perhaps psychotherapy, are the appropriate solutions to feelings of inadequacy and failed relationships, but breast implants are not.

The harm caused by implants is told in the horror stories of women who sought implants for trivial reasons or from motivations better served by other means. Despite their high hopes, the women suffered countless illnesses, severe pain, and multiple surgeries. Although a few brief alternate stories of reconstruction patients and happily augmented women were offered in the media reports, the horror story was most frequent and most elaborately told.

SAFETY

In addition to trivializing benefits and motives, the media accounts also presented reassurances of safety less powerfully than they did reports of harm. Safety accounts occupied a smaller amount of space than reports of illness. In addition, reassurances of safety were offered less often than were accounts of risk, danger, and side effects. Although nine tenths of newspaper, eight tenths of magazine, and half of television news segments linked side effects or risks to implants, only about a quarter of all news accounts featured a direct statement that breast implants were considered safe. Even then, the safety news was usually limited to only one or two lines of testimony or exposition, "Dow Corning believes in the safety of our products. . . . [Dow's spokesperson] said the company had committed millions of dollars to . . . make sure the products are safe" ("Breast Implant Maker," 1991, p. 11).

Other safety news reported denials of links between silicone implants and illness. One sixth of the implant stories included such dissociations. Most of these comments about the lack of causal links were only one line long. Typical is a statement from the Chief of Medicine at St. Thomas Hospital in Nashville, Tennessee, "There is no data implicating any defined or undefined systematic rheumatoid disease with breast implants" ("Panel Advises," 1992, p. 2A). Other medical testimony supported this argument, stating only "twenty-six patients of two million patients who have received breast implants have been reported in the literature as having connective tissue disease. This could easily be coincidental and not due to silicone breast implants" (Cruse, Novick, Brown, & Singer, 1991, p. 11A).

Usually the source of both types of safety claims was a plastic surgeon or an implant manufacturer. In the television news, every declaration of implant safety came from one of these sources. Audiences were likely to perceive a conflict of interest from both these sources. Compounding these credibility problems were the characterizations of plastic surgeons and implant manufacturers in news accounts. Chapter 7 focuses on the vilification of plastic surgeons in the print media. Chapter 8 highlights media attacks on Dow Corning Wright, the largest manufacturer of silicone implants.

In addition to the inclusion of direct safety claims and denials of causal relationships between implants and illness, the media accounts made attempts to qualify the risks. Although the news stories portrayed chronological links between silicone breast implants and side effects, they rarely drew direct causal connections unless the statements were attributed to women or their doctors. Usually the claims were qualified, as in this NBC lead-in, "Another disturbing medical story. . . . Cosmetic breast implants *may* cause disease" (Gould & Zucker, 1991a; italics added). The reports are full of references to "*possible* side effects" (Gross, 1991, p. A11; italics added), "*possible* dangers" (Mason, 1992, p. 3D; italics added), and "considerable reason to *suspect*" that "silicone causes cancers" (Rovner, 1991, p. 6; italics added).

Although news accounts qualify claims of dangers linked to silicone implants, print denials of causal links, and report safety claims, the narrative accounts of individual women's illnesses overwhelm these reassurances. News about health problems related to implants is reported much more often and in much more compelling forms than is safety news. The news audience is exposed to a media story that consistently draws a negative picture of silicone gel implants, despite its less frequent reassurances that most women have no problems.

CONCLUSION AND IMPLICATIONS

As Robert K. Manoff (1986) argued in *Reading the News*, "narratives are organizations of experience. They bring order to events by making them . . . make sense" (p. 228). Thus, the media's reliance on narrative as a way to convey implant risks and on testimony, exposition, and statistics to convey safety, dramatized the classic struggle between expert testimony and individual experience. The breast implant controversy was a "public moral argument" that relied on both a rational paradigm, with its references to expert testimony and scientific basis, and a narrative paradigm, which played out in the horror story, with experts, women with implants, and the society as a whole taking roles in the story (Fisher, 1984). The protagonists, the women with implants, were defined as the classic tragic heroines: destined for harm because of their tragic flaws of narcissism and pride. The proponents of safety were rational and abstract. Fisher argued that the narrative paradigm comes closer than the rational paradigm to explaining the world, because we rely on narratives ourselves to explain our everyday experiences. Thus, the narrative form of the media's coverage of the implant problems was more akin to the audience's own experiences. An attempt at identification through narrative compelled women to rely on the stories of other women for their knowledge and understanding of breast implants. The dramatic form describing implant danger was also powerful because it is more likely to be recalled. The news accounts that are most likely to be remembered are detailed narrative accounts of dangers told in dramatic terms (Singer & Endreny, 1993).

The compelling nature of the narrative form, its power to maintain attention, identification, and memory have implications for the audience's understanding of safety and risk. Women and physicians we interviewed referred to media as influential in multiple health decisions: whether to keep implants or have them removed, what kinds of implants women chose, and the types that doctors recommended. Relationships drawn in media stories between implants and illness were critical components in some women's diagnosis of silicone related diseases. Doctors justified unrestricted regulation of implants because of their benefits to women's emotional well-being following cancer surgery and to flat-chested women's newly found self-esteem following augmentation. The balance of benefit to harm is a stock issue in any decision about medical procedures and devices. Virtually no human activity is without risk of harm, but public awareness and perception of risks is influenced by media and can easily be incongruent with the actual probability of harm to the public (Singer & Endreny, 1993).

Several ideas from the study of such risk communication seem relevant to the media coverage about implants. First, it is easier to communicate about danger than about safety. Our media analysis confirms that far more attention is given to discussions of harm and side effects than to benefits and safety. Safety is expected; danger is unexpected. Thus, danger is news and safety is not. "Silicone Gel Implants Work Just Fine" was never a headline because implants were supposed to be effective. Women and doctors shared that expectation. The unexpected was presented in the media.

Second, danger makes dramatic stories. The accounts of women who believe their implants have made them ill are peopled with characters with human qualities whose lives have been altered. Conversely, the statistics about the large number of women without problems lacked a human dimension. Although we found the individual stories of satisfied women in chapter 4 to be compelling, and early media stories about mastectomy patients to be dramatic, these did not play out in media coverage during the controversy. Instead satisfied women were represented by statistics in the media; they were not fleshed out characters with whom others could identify.

Third, risks are more likely to be acceptable to people when the benefits are also clear. The news coverage speaks little of the benefits to patients and trivializes those on which it does elaborate. Missing are the compelling benefits from the women in chapter 4. In our interviews with women with implants, nearly all spoke positively of the significant benefits of the implants. Even those who came to believe that the implants were making them sick lamented the loss of self-esteem, normalcy, attractiveness, and femininity.

Yet the importance of those benefits did not find its way into the media stories during the height of the controversy. Breast cancer support groups did tell the FDA a benefit story, women face being disfigured or face dying from cancer. The availability of attractive implants gives them a choice that makes mastectomy more acceptable and, thus saves lives. Some mastectomy patients required implants to repair their ability to resume intimate relationships. Such stories appeared in the media a decade before the controversy:

> A Maryland woman, Patricia Gosselin, who had a mastectomy at 35, refused to let her husband look at her naked body for seven years; she wore her prosthesis and a bra even to bed. When she came home from the hospital with a newly constructed breast and showed it to her husband, she remembers, "his eyes filled with tears of joy. He just couldn't believe it. I feel as though I have been set free." (Seligman, 1980, p. 80)

In the absence of such stories, the FDA's ruling permitting postmastectomy use of gel implants may seem illogical. (If implants are a danger, shouldn't those who are ill be the first to be protected?) But when the power of the benefit advanced is considered, it is easy to understand the ruling. Over all, the mastectomy benefit was overwhelmed in the news coverage by the augmentation motives that were trivialized by the reports.

The public's ability to understand risks requires the awareness of both the problems and benefits associated with medical procedures and devices. The media's concentration on dangers and lack of attention to benefits is consistent with its treatment of other health hazards. The news media typically do not provide accounts of risks to be weighed, but focus on problems instead (Singer & Endreny, 1993). In the media treatment of breast implants, the difficulties were so often repeated and so varied, and the benefits so trivialized, that the risk seemed unacceptable.

The sheer amount of news coverage given to the breast implant story also heightens a perception of risk. Physicians and satisfied patients told us that the media had blown the controversy out of proportion to the actual number of women who were affected. One reason for the large amount of coverage may have been the population of women affected: "The media attend disproportionately to the risks of the more affluent . . . members of society" (Singer & Endreny, 1993, p. 43). Although more middle-income women are choosing implants, the devices are expensive, and augmentation is rarely covered by insurance. Consequently, the population of women who choose implants is likely to be well off financially. As a result, disproportionate attention may have been paid to breast implant hazards.

The small number of women affected has little relationship to the amount of media attention paid. Studies have revealed that the amount of news focused on a possible hazard appears to be unrelated to the number of people affected negatively. Indeed, the rarer hazards often receive more attention than the more common. Ordinary, everyday risks are accepted without question because they are so routine. Even aggregated small risks are not seen as dangerous compared to single dramatically portrayed risks. The dramatic, unusual, and unexpected nature of implant complications may be one reason why it received such a large amount of media coverage:

> The reason for the lack of congruence between the risk and the amount of media attention it receives lies in the man-bites-dog nature of news. A rare hazard is more newsworthy than a common one, other things being equal. A new hazard is more newsworthy than an old one. And a dramatic hazard—one that kills many people at once, suddenly or mysteriously—is more newsworthy than a long-familiar illness. (Singer & Endreny, 1993, p. 83)

Attention to rare and dramatic risks, such as the coverage of the implant dangers can lead readers to overestimate their occurrences. Singer and Endreny's (1993) survey of news stories and risk argued that the lack of correspondence between prevalence of a news story, and the number of people affected, creates an obstacle to the audience's accurate understanding of, and ability to weigh risks.

The dramatic portrayal of implant risks heightens the awareness and the perception of risk frequency. The dramatized risk seemed wholly avoidable because implants, not having been portrayed as having serious benefits, appeared trivial; only cosmetic. Implant surgery was portrayed as an avoidable dangerous procedure, one with dramatic unusual impact, and one without serious benefits.

The impact of the narrative portrayal of dangers, the trivialization and minimization of benefits, and the focus on rare problems appears to support physicians' claims that the media provided a compellingly negative perception of silicone breast implants. Tversky and Kahneman's 1973 study of toxic shock syndrome identified a similar media pattern, the selection of a hazard that was "relatively serious and relatively rare" (Singer & Endreny, 1993, p. 82). As a result, the public is likely to overestimate the likelihood of the harm's occurrence. In the case of toxic shock syndrome, a "notable public health threat, but a very rare one" caused significant changes in women's tampon-buying habits (Weiner, 1986, p. 158). Similarly, the FDA's restrictions on silicone implants may have preempted a public decline in the demand for implants, caused by the media accounts. Indeed, several women featured in chapter 4 chose saline implants before the moratorium or subsequent restrictions went into effect.

The negative perception of breast implants was encouraged by media accounts that dramatized harm, trivialized benefit, and emphasized danger over safety. Classic theories on news reporting concur that the media construct pictures of reality by the selection, arrangement, and emphasis placed on various elements of events (Altheide, 1974; Epstein, 1973; Tuchman, 1978). The narrative themes and focus of the news media implant story appear to be functions of the narrative paradigm and the constraints of news reporting on health risks, rather than a conspiracy against plastic surgeons, as our physician interviewees suggested. Nonetheless, the repetition of such stories in the news media can and did have powerful effects. Cultivation theory suggests that audiences who are repeatedly exposed to a consistent message will come to perceive the world through the media framework (Gerbner & Gross, 1976). Freimuth and Van Nevel (1981) related changes in awareness of risks to the amount of news coverage devoted to the subject. If these scholars are correct, the media coverage of silicone breast implants generally emerged as a frightening warning to women. The news coverage was not a balanced presentation of health information, but a narrative construction of the conclusion that implants were unsafe.

VILIFICATION STORIES:
PLASTIC SURGERY AND PROFIT[1]

We've [plastic surgeons] been the dog in the media for 10 years. They've done nothing but talk about us. But, you know, you can't make a pet out of a rattlesnake. (Tampa Bay Plastic Surgeon)

As we undertook the various studies reported in this book, it seemed that everywhere we looked we found plastic surgeons described as responsible for patients' distress. Yet, we had begun our work because several plastic surgeons had been determined to follow the highest ethical standards. We enjoyed the support of our faculty colleagues in plastic surgery and we had found them deeply concerned about patient well-being and the appropriate professional response to patient concerns. They were actively conducting research that might find a connection between silicone gel and illness if such a connection did indeed exist. Through their help, we were able to talk with numbers of plastic surgeons in community practice. Although all were troubled by the controversy and felt misunderstood, none seemed to wear horns and a tail. They talked about patients as we would want doctors to, with genuine concern and caring. They were troubled that patients who might benefit from gel implants could be denied the opportunity to choose them because of the political fallout from the controversy.

In the face of our experience with plastic surgeons, we began to wonder how to understand the strong negative image that had been assigned to them. Our survey data in chapter 9 showed that women, who relied only on the media for implant information, were more negative about implants and plastic surgeons than those who had talked to a doctor or nurse about the topic. We decided that a further analysis of media accounts, concentrating on the treatment of plastic surgeons, might be informative. Our analysis revealed that newspapers and magazines included characterizations of plastic surgeons as villains in the implant story. The impression has repercussions, not only for plastic surgeons, whose professionalism and credibility is placed in doubt, but also for perceptions of implant safety. As indicated in the previous chapter, the news media relied heavily on plastic surgeons' testimony to convey the message of implant safety, efficacy, and benefits. The physicians' credibility was essential to persuading the public

---

[1]An earlier version of this chapter was published in the *Journal of Plastic and Reconstructive Surgery*. This version is printed with permission from *JPRS*.

about minimal implant risks. Media accounts frequently undercut plastic surgeons' credibility by portraying them as antagonists in the women's horror stories, serving as poor sources of critical health care information and as incompetent physicians. In addition, plastic surgeons' credibility was decreased by media reports that depicted the medical community as divided in its assessment of breast implant health risks. Finally, plastic surgeons were cast in the role of business persons, whose motives were based on profit, not healing.

PLASTIC SURGEONS CAST IN THE ROLE OF ANTAGONISTS IN THE SICK PATIENTS "HORROR STORY"

The dominant theme of women's stories in the media was the horror story, a first person account of trauma and medical complications from women who believed their implants damaged their health. These narratives provided a base of identification with women, but often vilified doctors and implant manufacturers. In these news stories, heroines initially trusted surgeons who appeared to be skilled and caring. At first, patients believed the physicians' reassurances, but as the story progressed the patients encountered difficulties. Because the surgeons failed to provide adequate information about the risks of implants, women made bad decisions. The procedures that plastic surgeons performed resulted in pain, illness, and/or disfigurement for women patients. Betrayed by plastic surgeons they once trusted, women found peace and better health by disregarding the advice of experts. Although the plastic surgeons discussed in the various horror stories were different individuals, they shared two characteristics in the media accounts: (a) They failed to provide adequate health information to patients, and (b) they were inept surgeons; their work caused pain and disfigurement.

Plastic Surgeons' Failure to Provide Adequate Health Information

In their interaction with implant patients, plastic surgeons were frequently portrayed as failing to provide adequate health-related information, leading women to make decisions about implants they later regretted. In some stories physicians failed to tell patients about safety risks; in others they misinformed women. Alternative accounts described plastic surgeons who did not obtain enough information about the patients to give good advice.

Repeatedly, women patients stated that their physicians had failed to inform them about possible side effects and health risks during initial visits. Karen Koskoff indicated that she was "too busy beating breast cancer to question implant safety" when she decided to have reconstructive surgery, "No one told me there were risks" ("What Price," 1992, p.16). Another patient indicated that her plastic surgeon "did not mention the possibility of complete loss of sensation in the breasts" (Eagan, 1992, p. 124).

Although most of the accounts focus on plastic surgeons' omissions, some narratives characterized physicians as overtly misinforming patients:

Even before the reports of autoimmune diseases, surgeons probably knew that silicone implants were likely to cause capsular contracture. They also probably knew that the implants might rupture, leaking silicone in to the body. . . ."My surgeon told me, 'You could jump off the Empire State Building, and you'd be dead, but the implants would be intact,'" recalls Barbara Johnston. . . . Two years later, when her right implant ruptured, her surgeon, who is certified by the American Board of Plastic Surgery, assured her that she was "the first woman in history ever to have this problem." (Eagan, 1992, p. 125)

In 1984, reports of ruptured implants were available to plastic surgeons. One concludes from the story that the physician was either ignorant of fundamental facts about the procedure he performed, or was lying to the patient. Either conclusion undermines his credibility as a medical adviser.

Even women who directly asked their physicians about the risks frequently reported that plastic surgeons skirted the issue or minimized the problems, "I asked if there were any dangers. He said that about 10 percent of women who have implants develop hardness" (Jones, 1992, p. 59). When the patient developed capsular contraction following her surgery she did her own research and concluded, "It turned out that hardness is very common—and my doctor was wrong when he told me in 1981 that only 10 percent get it" (Jones, 1992, p. 59). Another patient asked, "Is this safe?" Her plastic surgeon replied, "Let me put it this way . . . both my wife and daughter have implants, and I'm not worried" (Mithers, 1992, p. 84). When Nancy Falbo inquired about possible links between illness and implants, "the doctors brainwashed me into thinking it couldn't be the implants" (Ripley, 1992, p. 6B).

The women's accounts of interactions with their physicians often included scenes in which physicians spent too little time with them to give good medical advice. One patient visited her plastic surgeon, concerned that her implant had ruptured. "He spent less than two minutes examining me, then assured me that everything was fine." A subsequent visit to another plastic surgeon revealed that the implants had ruptured and had been leaking for years (Sanders, 1992, p. 22). Another young woman seeking initial information on implants reported that "The young plastic surgeon, after a brief glance at my A-cup-sized breasts, assured me that I was a 'perfect candidate' for silicone implants. . . . and promised me that there were virtually no risks to this procedure" (Eagan, 1992, p. 124). Still another woman reported that her plastic surgeon "prods my chest for ten seconds, then pronounces the tissue healthy enough for surgery" (Mithers, 1992, p. 84). The accounts emphasized the small amount of time that plastic surgeons spent with patients before advising the women about their risks or health. The cumulative impression of such scenes is that physicians did not have adequate information on which to base their diagnoses. According to these accounts, women were misled by their plastic surgeons into believing their implants were or would be trouble free. Instead, as indicated in chapter 6, the women patients reported multiple problems and debilitating diseases.

Plastic Surgeons As Inept Practitioners

Many of the horror stories portrayed plastic surgeons as incompetent physicians whose operations and medical advice proved unsuccessful. Plastic surgeons' promises and reassurances were followed by multiple and severe medical complications. Sybil Goldrich reported that she "interviewed three reputable plastic surgeons . . . each assured her that the procedure would be simple with very little risk involved" (Regush, 1992, p. 25). Following her implant surgery, Goldrich developed infections, and within 2 months her breasts were "hard as rocks" (Regush, 1992, p. 25). Within 2 years, Goldrich had endured five painful surgeries without correcting the problems. Some plastic surgeons were depicted as careless and reckless with patient safety. A caller to a patient hot line "told of a doctor who removed her polyurethane-covered breast implants—the kind being investigated for possible links to cancer—washed them off and *put them back in*" (James, 1992, p. 1D). Another plastic surgeon reportedly "allowed his bookkeeper to administer general anesthesia during an office surgery. The patient died" (Scheer, 1991b, p. A28).

The stories also depict plastic surgeons as promising much, but delivering little. Multiple problems and unresolved complaints are common in the news accounts. The following is a typical saga:

> A plastic surgeon . . . told her it was a simple operation and assured her she'd be happy with the results,"Eight months later my left breast got as hard as a rock. My doctor said not to worry, the hardness would go away. When it didn't, he suggested vigorously massaging my breasts daily. When that didn't work, he told me 'some better implants' had been developed. So I agreed to a second surgery. Two months later my breasts became congested and painful. The doctor said that I had probably developed an infection and that the implants would have to be temporarily removed. After my third surgery to clear up the infection, I noticed that the infected breast had shrunk down so that it was smaller than before I had implants, and it was an odd, twisted shape. Even after a fourth implant surgery, my breasts remained totally different in size and shape. Then they both hardened." (Nashner & White, 1977, pp. 53-54)

At every turn, the plastic surgeon's suggestions and diagnoses fail to provide a solution to the woman's problems, until at last, she is worse off than before her augmentation or reconstruction. The plastic surgeon is seen through the patient's eyes as a source of false promises and medical incompetence.

Plastic Surgeons As Combatants in a Medical Community Divided in its Assessment of Health Risks

Print media accounts described a medical community in conflict over breast implant complications, safety, and restrictions. In the midst of the controversy, plastic surgeons repeatedly stated that silicone implants were safe and that the vast majority of women were happy with reconstruction and augmentation. Condemning the anecdotal substance of challenges to implant safety, most plastic surgeons were quoted in news accounts indicating that there was no scientific evidence of risk. Yet, the media accounts placed their adamant claims of safety within a larger scene of medical and historical controversy, giving the impression that plastic surgeons may not have been supported by the medical community at large, nor by a historical track record of medical risks associated with breast implants.

The stories featured plastic surgeons as major combatants in that drama. "Furious" over the restrictions on implants, the plastic surgeons were "ready to do battle" with the FDA (Seligman, Hager, & Springen, 1992, p. 67). Stories suggested that surgeons were powerful players having "amassed a $4 million war chest to keep implants [unrestricted]" (Vick, 1991, p. 3A) and used the voice of the influential American Society of Plastic and Reconstructive Surgery (ASPRS) to make its case: "The ASPRS assures prospective customers that 'breast implants are among the safest surgically implanted devices in use today'" ("Booming Busts," 1991, p. 81). Media accounts reminded readers of the enduring commitment made by plastic surgeons to implants: "Plastic surgeons have long maintained that implants are both necessary and safe" (Rovner, 1991, p. 6). The physicians denied the existence of any disease related to implants: "Though they support continuing research, most plastic surgeons dispute that silicone-associated disease exists" (James, 1991, p. 10F).

The narratives depicted the majority of plastic surgeons as adamantly supporting the efficacy and safety of implants. Yet, the media placed the surgeons in opposition to other members of the medical and scientific community, "No wonder the process [of determining safety] has been so agonizing. The debate over the safety of breast implants has set doctors against each other" (Seligman & Church, 1992, p. 75). Physicians and scientists were "divided over the risks" associated with silicone leaks (Fischer, 1991, p. 98). The stories described women who suffered diverse illnesses "now attributed by some doctors to their implants. . . . meanwhile, plastic surgeons and implant manufacturers pooh-poohed the whole thing" (James, 1992, p. 2D). The media reflected the division between plastic surgeons and rheumatologists over the identification of implant-related autoimmune disease:

> [At FDA hearings many doctors] complained . . . that most of the material presented to them has been anecdotal rather than scientific. . . . [But] doctors treating patients shown on the slides told the panel that they suspected the implants as the cause of the trouble and that, in some cases, when the devices were removed the problems either went away or stabilized. ("Panel Advises," 1992, p. 2A)

Media accounts also placed plastic surgeons in opposition to radiologists who feared the implications of implants on the ability to make early diagnoses of breast cancer:

> Another thing that worried the expert witnesses [at the FDA hearings] is that, if implants are in place, screening of breasts using x-rays is less likely to detect a cancer when it is still small and potentially most curable. The plastic-surgery society disputes this, and says that the implants can sometimes make breast tumors easier to find. The American College of Radiologists disagrees. ("Booming Busts," 1991, p. 81)

The media showed plastic surgeons at odds with other medical professionals in the assessment of risks related to the breast implants. Beyond this, the accounts invited the audience to compare contemporary surgeons' safety claims with a historical litany of problems related to augmentation and reconstruction: "Some surgeons have long recognized the potential dangers of silicone and sought alternatives" (Eagan, 1992, p. 126). Reports dating back decades were listed as among the warning signs that implants had health risks: "As early as the 1970s, Dow Corning managers and several plastic surgeons who installed the devices had disclosed their concerns about the product's safety" (Byrne, 1992, p. 33). Other reports dated the problems back to the 1960s: "Since silicone breast implants were introduced in the 1960s, many questions have been raised of their safety" (Purvis, 1991, p. 70). When Dow Corning was accused of hiding safety hazards from the public, one article reported:

> In numerous memos from the mid-1970s, Dow Corning employees said the gel bleed and the implant ruptures were the top complaint of surgeons who inserted the devices. . . . Since as early as 1971, the documents showed, plastic surgeons and even company officials periodically have warned that the soft envelopes of gel . . . can break and their silicone filling leak out . . . into surrounding tissue. ("Memos Show Problems," 1992, p. 2A)

The plastic surgeons' safety claims are set against not only historical questions about safety, but past reassurances by surgeons about implant safety, which were later found to be false. Several magazines and newspapers printed extensive histories of augmentation and reconstruction procedures during the silicone controversy. These accounts reminded the reader that plastic surgeons had recommended numerous procedures that turned out to be harmful, for example, preventive mastectomies, closed capsulotomies, silicone injections, and Natural Y implants.

One of the most compelling reversals concerned preventative or prophylactic mastectomies. The stories included plastic surgeons' advice to women with family or personal histories of breast cancer. Given a high likelihood of cancer, some plastic surgeons recommended preventive mastectomies and reconstruction with implants. After one woman's right breast mastectomy, her plastic surgeon suggested that she have her left breast removed "to prevent the possible development of cancer on that side." The magazine reported that subsequently, "Such 'preventative' surgery . . . is highly controversial, and many breast surgeons believe it is unnecessary at best" (Eagan, 1992, p. 125). Other reports told of plastic surgeons who routinely recommended closed capsulotomy as a treatment for hardening of the implants. During the procedure the plastic surgeon vigorously applies pressure to the hardened tissue surrounding the implant, manually breaking the scar tissue. Subsequently, media reported, "This procedure . . . can be excruciatingly painful and carries the risk of popping the implant along with the scar tissue; the FDA now recommends that this procedure not be performed" (Eagan, 1992, p. 124). Promises and problems with earlier forms of implants were also included in media coverage during the controversy over silicone implants. The Même implant and its precursor, the Natural Y were featured as devices heralded by plastic surgeons as solutions to problems with previous implants. Placed in thousands of women, the media described multiple complications. In the early 1970s, the developers of Natural Y promised "total fixation . . . no deep tissue ingrowth . . . [it] reduces . . . fibrous encapsulation" (Nashner & White, 1977, p. 85). The Natural Y became popular with plastic surgeons, but within 3 years, the usual scar tissue formed:

> By 1975, Ashley's "Natural Y" was not only hardening but causing foreign-body reactions. [Physicians at] Vanderbilt University School of Medicine reported finding particles of polyurethane scattered throughout the tissues of five patients, as the wall of the implant slowly began to disintegrate, just as the old sponge-type implant did 20 years earlier. . . . in 1973 researchers found "a definite and significant foreign-body reaction" to polyurethane implants in rabbits. (Nashner & White, 1977, p. 85)

Subsequently, the Même implant was designed and prescribed to prevent the problems inherent in the Natural Y device. Subsequent media reports included statements by scientists questioning the safety of these improved devices:

> Kossovsky, an assistant professor of pathology and laboratory medicine at UCLA School of Medicine, who for 14 years has studied the interactions between body tissues and implants. . . . notes. . . . "If you were picking a material to put in the body and you wanted it to break down, you could hardly come up with a better candidate [than the coating found on Même implants]."

> Though Kossovsky and others believe the behavior of polyurethane in the body should have been predicted long ago, it was only recently that the material's behavior aroused widespread concern. (Weiss, 1991, p. 1060)

The media portrayed the development of implants as a series of missteps in which devices were used before they were properly tested. Reassurances were made about safety and efficacy, and then retracted when problems arose. The portrayal provided a picture of long-term uncertainty within the medical community about the safety and risk associated with implants. One plastic surgeon "believes much too little is known about the risks of both polyurethane and leaking silicone gel. 'We're just not sure of the full implications, just as with an oil spill'" (Seligmann, Yoffe, & Hager, 1991, p. 56). Media created an image of a scientific community "scrambling to determine the level of risks associated with the implants" (Weiss, 1991, p. 1060). In the portrayal of experts disagreeing, the unqualified, staunch claims of safety from the majority of plastic surgeons seemed doubtful and self-serving especially given the motives attributed to the group.

Plastic Surgeons Cast As Profit-Oriented Businesspersons

In the first two narrative themes, physicians were portrayed as interacting with patients and as players within the medical controversy. A third narrative theme focused on the plastic surgeons' motives for misinforming women and advocating implant safety in the face of the health controversy. Those depictions focused on the profit motives and businesslike setting surrounding plastic surgery.

News stories often attributed profit motives to plastic surgeons: "For three decades, America's breast obsession has enabled surgeons and chemical companies to turn bags of silicone putty into gold" (Cowley, Springen, & Hager, 1992, p. 56). One magazine writer explained that the surgeons' resistance to the FDA restrictions on silicone implants is based on "the loss of a substantial and lucrative part of their practices" (Seligman, Hager, & Springen, 1992, p. 67). Other news reports highlighted the high salaries of plastic surgeons, explaining: "Plastic surgeons are among the highest paid group of doctors. According to *Medical Economics* magazine, their median income in 1989, the latest figures available, was $211,250" (Craddock, 1992, p. 2B). One report claimed that plastic surgeons hid risks from patients to protect the physicians' incomes:

> If the public had been warned years ago of the vast array of illnesses linked to breast implants, wouldn't . . . the plastic surgeons have noted "decreased revenue" as a direct result? It seems that all along this has been the primary concern, when it should have been the health of the women involved. (McMahon, 1992, p. 2)

Congruent with the profit motive, stories about physicians focused on actions more appropriate for corporate America than for Marcus Welby. Physicians are depicted as promoting their businesses rather than healing the sick:

> About 750,000 women a year elect to have cosmetic surgery, spurred on by ubiquitous images of the body beautiful . . . and by doctors' newspaper ads. . . . In Houston last March, plastic surgeon Dr. Franklin Rose took out an ad in the *Houston Chronicle*, explaining that the "cultural influence is such in this city that for a woman to feel attractive usually includes a Mercedes, a gold Rolex, and three or four operations—nose, breasts, liposuctions. It's just part of living in this city in a certain way, in a certain socioeconomic strata." The ad ends like this: "The Texas woman is a combination of many things, not the least of which is a surgeon's scalpel" (Regush, 1992, p. 26).

The scene in which plastic surgeons operate was compared to a business designed to produce profit. News reports focused on plastic surgery as a "big business": "Breast augmentation is a $450-million-a-year business" (Regush, 1992, p. 26). Another report indicated that breast implants were a "300 million U. S. industry" (Seligman, Hager, & Springen, 1992, p. 67). Plastic surgeons were described as part of an "aggressive medical industry that appears to be driven by a gold rush fever" (Scheer, 1991b, p. A29).

Specific stories highlighted a "marketing atmosphere" in plastic surgeons' offices. One patient said her initial visit to a Los Angeles plastic surgeon was:

> . . . like entering the showroom of Breasts 'R' Us. In one corner stands a small bronze figurine of a Native American maiden, her chest thrust forward aggressively, nipples erect. On a wall, Venus emerges naked from the sea in a reproduction of Botticelli's painting. Reading matter includes a powder-blue brochure in which 16 different women bare their chest—both before and after their implant surgery. Before my eyes, small breasts bloom into big, bigger, or *huge* ones. Here at the Breast Enhancement Medical Center, big breasts are big business. (Mithers, 1992, p. 83)

Plastic surgeons' offices were described as "businesses where 'credit cards [are] accepted, [and] financing [is] available'" (Mithers, 1992, p. 84). Some magazine articles feature the "top dollar" deposits that plastic surgeons required "up front" from $1,525 in Omaha to $5,300 in New York City (Fischer, 1991, p. 97).

The cumulative impression was that plastic surgeons are profit, rather than health, oriented in need of "more incentive to pay as much attention to safety as profitability" ("More Action," 1992, p. 8A). Their actions included hiding information from patients, minimizing health risks, and performing ineffective and sometimes harmful procedures in order to fulfill profit motives. The adamant and active stand they took in the medical controversy over implants seemed at odds with other subspecialties and less than certain in a scientific community attempting to establish the actual level of risk.

CREDIBILITY AND THE MEDIA PORTRAYAL
OF PLASTIC SURGEONS

What are the implications of these characterizations? One of the most serious is the lowered credibility of plastic surgeons as sources of information in the breast implant controversy, and a consequent increase in credibility of the women who presented them as antagonists.

Classic theories of public credibility suggest that for one to be believed, one must be perceived to be of goodwill, caring for the well-being of others more than one's own self-interest. In addition, one must be perceived to be of good character: honest, generous, and just. Finally, believable sources are those who are experts. They have up-to-date and accurate knowledge and are willing to share it (Golden, Berquist, & Coleman, 1989, pp. 523–534). Media characterizations of plastic surgeons paint pictures of individuals who fail to measure up to these credibility tests.

Professionals are agents for others, employed because of their superior knowledge and/or skill. The professional accepts the obligation to represent well the one who has engaged her. But one can be an ineffective agent, perform incompetently or carelessly. In so doing, credibility based on expertise is undermined. If a surgeon performs surgery poorly, lacks knowledge that would be expected, or is criticized by other physicians, the surgeon's expertise, and consequently credibility, come into question. The stories of repeated surgeries, leaking or ruptured implants, and physicians having to undo the mistakes of others undermine credibility in that way.

In addition to being an inexpert agent, one can also be an unethical agent by failing to give primacy to the client's (patient's) interests. Here the idea of goodwill is the key. Goodwill demands that one subordinate self-concern to concern for the other (Aristotle, 1932, pp. 92, 118–119). Of all the professions, medicine carries with it, perhaps along with the ministry, the highest expectation for unselfishness, even self-sacrifice at times. But surgeons who engage in opulent display, charge large fees payable up front, use high-pressure sales pitches, spend little time with patients, and avoid responsibility for poor outcomes, fail to meet our expectation of goodwill. All these actions do indeed appear in the media stories.

They suggest violation of the ethic of agency common to all professionals. The lawyer who designs a client's will to maximize rather than minimize probate expenses, especially lawyer fees is violating the agency ethic. The politician who is more influenced by lobbyists' favors than constituents' needs fails to follow the ethic of agency. The cleric who exploits vulnerable members of the flock for financial gain or sexual satisfaction has failed to be an ethically responsible agent. When a physician acts as an agent for a patient and is paid for that service, it is unethical for that physician to act from self-interest rather than from patient interest. If the plastic surgeon is believed to be more interested in making money than in patients' well-being, then the surgeon will be regarded as an unethical agent. When the stories about implants in the news media recast the doctor–patient relationship into a buyer-seller relationship, with the buyer needing to beware, the credibility of the plastic surgeon, portrayed and, by extension, of other plastic surgeons, is sapped.

If plastic surgeons also appear in the published stories to be willing to lie, to hide information, and to ignore patients when surgery turns out badly, the damage to credibility from poor expertise and the lack of goodwill be compounded by the absence of good character. Plastic surgeons will not be the "good guys" doctors are supposed to be. They will be seen as not knowing what they are doing and as untrustworthy. The higher level of behavior we expect from doctors, as opposed to other professions, makes the problem worse. The fall from grace has been farther and harder because the physician's pedestal is taller.

At this point, it seems reasonable to ask whether the stories in the media had the damaging impact on the image of plastic surgeons that we suggest. We have access to no comprehensive study of public perceptions about plastic surgeons' credibility, but we can look to our own public opinion survey reported in chapter 9, which indicates that those who relied only on the media for information were less favorable toward physicians than those who had also talked to a doctor or a nurse. We also know from that study that those respondents who had implants or knew someone with implants were more favorable to implants on a number of items than were respondents who reported only media sources of information. These tendencies are consistent with our conversations with members of the public generally who believe the horror stories rather than the rational discourse of the experts. The plastic surgeons we have talked with almost universally feel misrepresented, misunderstood, and devalued by society.

Plastic surgeons are represented in the media coverage as characters who violate our expectation of the way physicians are supposed to be. These medical professionals do not fit the archetype of caring doctor: concerned, compassionate, patient, and selfless. But do readers believe these accounts? The data in chapter 9 suggest that they do. Here two concepts may be helpful: narrative fidelity and narrative probability. *Narrative fidelity* refers to whether a story fits our understanding of what the world is like. *Narrative probability* refers to a story's coherence with other accounts (Fisher, 1984).

The portrayal of plastic surgeons may be believable to the extent that it fits the reader's personal experiences. Research on patients' attitudes toward contemporary medical practice is sobering. The recently developed marketing strategies that undergird medical profits have become a visible part of public concern and discourse (Todd, 1989). The public seems overwhelmingly convinced that the medical system, even the way doctors practice, needs to be reformed. Patients report routinely experiencing frustration with physicians due to mistaken diagnoses and doctors' perceived lack of concern (Korsch, Gozzi, & Francis, 1968; Korsch & Negrete, 1972; Mechanic, 1968). A survey of research on patient dissatisfaction with medical care reveals patients' "demoralization." Patients believe "their own views were ignored" by physicians (Todd, 1989, p. 18). Patients have developed new desires for involvement in discussions and decisions about their own care (American Board of Family Practice, 1987; Harris & Associates, 1982). Yet many doctors view such discussions as too time consuming to be permitted, and patients complain that doctors do not spend enough time with them. Of some comfort may be the fact that patients' attitudes toward their own physicians are generally more positive than their attitudes toward the profession generally (American Board of Family Practice, 1987). Yet, the stories they read on this topic are not about their own physicians; most Americans have not visited a plastic surgeon.

Even if readers' own experiences with physicians have been positive, they may have heard about problems from friends or family members as well as read about them in the media. Those accounts may include problems like those described by implant patients. If so, the breast implant stories may ring true. They fit the world as the readers understand it. They have significant narrative fidelity.

However, the news accounts violate other aspects of reader expectations. Because they are inconsistent with most traditional stories about doctors, they create inconsistency in our image of physicians. Physicians are not supposed to be business-like. They are supposed to be caring, informing professionals who put their patients' concerns before their own. The impious media portrayal of plastic surgeons challenges our traditional assumptions and beliefs about the medical profession. The media stories that are incongruent with the traditional physician image are at odds with narrative probability. One way to handle the psychological tension created by the inconsistency between these two cognitions is to regard plastic surgeons as different from other doctors who would not act as the press says plastic surgeons do. That separation comes at the expense of the positive image of plastic surgery. Plastic surgeons become different from the competent caring doctors of other physician stories. Narrative probability can be reinforced by denying to plastic surgeons the positive images contained in traditional stories of good doctors.

Problems in Dealing With the Conflict in Underlying Societal Values

Compounding the perceived division between doctors and plastic surgeons is considerable social ambivalence about our culture's attitudes toward physical appearance. Images are the business of plastic surgeons. They help patients by improving patients' appearances. The training, diligence, and skill that the profession brings to bear on patients' image problems are formidable. In applying these skills, plastic surgeons work minor miracles compared to the state of the art just a few years ago. Yet, in a way unique to their specialty, plastic surgeons face an image problem of their own. Despite the virtuosity with which it is performed, plastic surgery is not always regarded as serious medicine. Even though the evidence is strong that plastic surgery improves patients' lives and that patients are glad they underwent the procedures, much plastic surgery is not considered central enough to the healing arts to be included under health insurance reimbursement schemes. "Surely, if it were real medicine, Blue Cross would pay for it!" critics remark. Facelifts for Phyllis Diller, enlarged breasts for Dolly Parton, and nose jobs and tummy tucks for the country club set do not fit the model of either Marcus Welby or Albert Schweitzer. As a result, plastic surgeons are all too often viewed as working at the periphery of medicine, pandering to the vanity of the rich rather than helping to cure human suffering. The news stories about trivial benefits for breast augmentation found in chapter 6 reinforce the plastic surgeons' marginalization.

Into this milieu comes the plastic surgeon, devoted to making a difference in appearance. Our conflict over the value of appearance becomes focused on what plastic surgeons do. Everyone applauds when surgery makes the accident victim's face look normal again or corrects a cleft palate. However, we ridicule those who believe they can make themselves beautiful or young through cosmetic surgery.

In the movie *Doc Hollywood*, which played nationally during the controversy, a resident chides the protagonist about his plan to become a plastic surgeon, "I thought you were going to practice real medicine." The justification recited by the Hollywood plastic surgeon he wants to join, played appropriately enough by George Hamilton, rationalizes that the profits from the various enhancements of the rich make possible needed work on the poor. But the litany rings hollow, when spoken in the plastic surgeon's opulent office, as he gives patients only cursory attention and seems most interested in his golf game. The hero finds redemption by renouncing plastic surgery for "real" medicine, family practice in a small rural town, and true love. We walk out of the movie house past slick posters for coming attractions, elaborate plastic facades, and oversized boxes containing undersized quantities of nutritionally barren sweets, reassured that substance does really matter and mere cosmetics are superficial. How can plastic surgeons expect admiration in a society deeply conflicted about the values underlying much of what they do?

Problems in Dealing With the Press

The key to the maintenance of the plastic surgeon's professional image is the expression of traditional physician values of compassion and helping others. But the media coverage of the implant controversy did not attribute those motives to plastic surgeons. Instead, doctors were portrayed as more interested in money than in patients. The media did not tell stories of how hard doctors had tried to help patients, of their disappointments when things did not go well, or of times when they had gone to great lengths to make things right for patients. Chapter 5 includes such stories from plastic surgeons that might have appeared in the press. One doctor we interviewed talked about the long search to find a material that would give good results to women who wanted larger breasts and reconstructions. He described early attempts with other materials and explained how pleased he had been when silicone gel implants became available, because they were so much better than earlier implants. Chapter 5 details plastic surgeons' attempts to contact and reassure women patients. Such stories describe long-term concern for patients and do much to refute the impression that plastic surgeons are only concerned about money, but they did not appear in the press during the controversy. The result was that the evidence of good character and goodwill that could have enhanced plastic surgeons' credibility did not make it into the papers.

We suspect that plastic surgeons did not feel comfortable telling their stories to reporters. Our interviews with plastic surgeons revealed deep-seated distrust of news media. When the physicians were asked about reporters, the doctors characterized the media as detrimental to plastic surgeons' image, and, perhaps, to the truth: "I think the media . . . have been very biased. I mean if you see a victim, a patient who's on TV, who has a problem, who's a mess. And then you see this rich plastic surgeon in his thousand dollar suit . . . sitting there. Who are you going to feel sorry for?"

Our interviewees described the press coverage as sensational attempts to sell papers or raise Nielsen ratings rather than present the facts accurately. They explained that many of their patients called for reassurance after the media coverage became intense. The 1990 Connie Chung special and 1991 replay on CBS was cited repeatedly as generating patient concern:

Well, first of all everybody called me and said, "Did you see those green, slimy, dripping implants on television?" . . . Frankly the patients came in anxious, but came in with no symptoms. They were just worried. They just wanted to know if they were OK. The media hype became so repetitive and strident that I think all of them felt compelled to talk to their doctor.

The press received little respect from our plastic surgeon interviewees. Not only did they believe that the press distorted the facts, but that distortion is what one should expect from the news media. One physician compared the disastrous effects of media coverage about Audi automobiles to the future of silicone implants. He referred to a presentation on the danger of the Audi 5000 carried on *60 Minutes*:

You've not heard Ed Bradley on *60 Minutes* saying, "Gee, I'm sorry we made this terrible mistake." You've not heard a single television or newspaper program say, "Gosh this was all a giant mistake and we're sorry we ruined Audi's business." . . . Well the same thing's going to happen with silicone gel.

Another interviewee expressed even longer term distrust of the media: "We've been the dog in the media for 10 years. They've done nothing but talk about us. But, you know, you can't make a pet out of a rattlesnake. And that's been proven once again."

If plastic surgeons do not trust the media to present stories accurately even if given good information, then plastic surgeons are not likely to want to talk to reporters. If they do talk to reporters, they are likely to keep their comments limited to what surgeons see as the relevant facts. But those facts are part of the rational paradigm expressed in statistics and expert testimony, not the dramatic, compelling narratives told by members of Command Trust or the Silicone Sisters. Indeed, as indicated in chapter 6, the rational discourse was used to present implant safety in news accounts.

Communicating safety requires the generation of compelling human stories of safety and benefit. A few detailed stories of dramatic emotional transformations for mastectomy patients were printed in magazines before 1991. Only a few fragments of such accounts appeared between 1990 and 1992. The stories of satisfied women described in chapter 4 were also absent. We suspect that they were not often presented to reporters. Because plastic surgeons, like many other professionals, have been distrustful of the press, they may have attempted to avoid reporters fearing misquotation. Plastic surgeons are also likely to have found the rational discourse of statistics and expert testimony persuasive to themselves, and repeated it to reporters. That is what shows up in the stories, but it also has less impact than the dramatic narratives of risk leading to harm for suffering people.

Our study of media accounts showed that plastic surgeons were not presented in the press coverage as people with human dimensions. They did not have hopes, dreams, or frustrations. They did not have families, ambitions, or hobbies. Instead they were one-dimensional figures whose description came only from their critics.

Similarly, their motives were imputed by their adversaries, not by the doctors themselves. Doctors were not described as acting to help patients or to further knowledge of the problem. Such descriptions were found in physicians' accounts and in the stories of satisfied women. The narratives would have implied positive motives, but they were absent. Some of the stories were interesting enough and dramatic enough to grab attention. They would have made good copy.

Given that the press made attempts to cover all sides of the controversy, surely, the balancing would have included such stories, not just the rational material, if reporters had been given them. One reporter who covered this story told us that she had heard dramatic stories of problems from so many women that she had come to believe that there was a real risk. The women who had horror stories to tell were aggressive in telling them and contacting her. Even with this belief, the stories she wrote attempted to balance the coverage. What might have happened if more plastic surgeons had called and told her stories of their experiences? Of course, that would have required a trust in the press not evident in our interviews. The coverage, then, affirmed plastic surgeons' expectations and the prophecy became self-fulfilling.

This lack of balance in what reporters wrote could easily have created an exposure bias. Few or no women called the reporter just mentioned to say they were doing fine. If plastic surgeons, uncertain of the fairness of reporters, also provided little input, reporters could easily have concluded that the frequency of problems was great and that there was the clear connection between implants and illness that the complaining callers asserted. Surely, the preponderance of risks and side effects reported in chapter 6 reflects such perceptions.

At the same time, reluctance to talk to the press runs counter to what is, perhaps, the strongest value held by reporters: access. Their whole function is dependent on gaining access to information and opinion. Reporters lobby for open governmental processes, defend the confidentiality of sources even from prison, and badger people they believe are newsworthy for comments because of the centrality of access to reportorial success. When an individual does not return a call or make a comment, the reporter will often say, "Dr. Jones failed to return our call," or "Ms. Cortez refused to comment," implying in both cases that the refuser has something to hide. If plastic surgeons avoided the press, reporters quite naturally would have found it difficult to be sympathetic, just as many physicians find it difficult to be sympathetic to the noncompliant patients who frustrate what doctors see as their essential function.

Problems in the Professional Practice Itself

Although we did not set out to be critics of others' professional practice, we could not do the amount of study we have done without coming to feel that some of the damage to the image of plastic surgery as a profession may be created by what some plastic surgeons actually do or fail to do. It is difficult to argue that the "Breasts 'R' Us" example presented previously represents patient-centered medicine at its best.

The stories of patients receiving cursory examinations before being told they need implants make us uncomfortable. The stories of patients rejected by doctors, or of doctors' unwillingness to listen to patients, may have been exaggerated, but even if only partly true, point to less concern for patient well-being than we would hope to find in our own physicians. The general aura of wealth and the suggestion of greed surrounding cosmetic surgery seems a poor fit with the ideal of medicine that serves, rather than profits from, patients.

Any profession must tolerate some degree of variability in the way practitioners exercise their art. Those at the extreme can be tolerated as long as they are seen as aberrant, not typical. In the media portrayal of plastic surgery what we hope are extreme practices were presented as representative. Can the profession afford to tolerate the current range of extremes? What constraints might be reasonable and enforceable? These questions should be dealt with seriously by the profession itself, for there is the possibility that some of the negative impact on the image of plastic surgery has been generated by press depictions that are, in part, accurate.

In Florida, we have watched organized medicine fail in political action when the public saw its efforts as aimed at protecting doctors' pocketbooks more than protecting patient's well-being. A statewide referendum to place a lower cap on malpractice awards by juries was soundly defeated. Despite resistance from the Florida Medical Association, the Florida Legislature placed severe restrictions on physician ownership of imaging facilities and the like. This law came on the heels of publication of research showing that doctor-owned centers charged higher fees and that the doctors who owned them were more likely to refer patients for imaging. As we contemplate the response of organized medicine to health care reform in the United States, we wonder whether doctors as a whole, or at least certain specialty groups, are not in danger of seeming more concerned with their own financial position in the health care system than with how patients are cared for.

There is an important lesson in what happened to plastic surgeons as a result of the implant controversy. So long as doctors are viewed as primarily committed to their patients' well-being, they will be admired and listened to. When they appear to be self-serving, whether they are, or whether the media images fail to include the stories of their concern for patients, they will be vilified and lose their credibility.

8

VILIFICATION STORIES:
THE FALL OF DOW CORNING

Tonja E. Olive

> The most important battle to be fought is not in a court of law. It's in the court of public opinion. That's the key lesson gleaned from James Burke's deft handling of Johnson & Johnson's Tylenol crisis. Accept responsibility. Forget short-term profitability. As Gerald Meyers, a professor at Carnegie Mellon University's business school, puts it: "If you win public opinion, the company can move forward and get through it. If you lose there, it won't make any difference what happens in a court of law." (Byrne, 1992, p. 33)

As the media heightened awareness of the controversy surrounding silicone breast implants, manufacturers struggled to maintain public confidence and government approval for their products. Dow Corning Wright, a joint venture between Dow Chemical and Corning, was the largest manufacturer of silicone breast implants and had been a pioneer in their design since the 1960s. An estimated 450,000 to 1,300,000 American women have Dow Corning implants (Reibstein, Washington, Tsaintor, & Hager, 1992, p. 38; Walker, 1992, p. 1A). Controlling 30% of the implant market, Dow Corning led McGhan Medical Corporation, Bioplasty Inc., Mentor Corporation, and Bristol-Meyers Squibb. Throughout the decades of its market leadership Dow Corning had affirmed the safety and efficacy of its implants.

But, by April 1992, the company's actions belied its safety claims. Dow Corning, beset by hundreds of legal suits, withdrew from the implant market. Although less than 1% of its almost $2 billion sales came from implants, some estimates placed Dow's potential liability at $2 billion in legal settlements ("Dow to Stop," 1992, p. 5A; "Analysts," 1992, p. 6A). By the time Dow Corning withdrew from the market in 1992, the company had pledged $10 million to new safety tests, the establishment of an advisory "woman's council," and the development of a registry to follow women with implants. In addition, the manufacturer had promised to pay $1,200 for the removal of its implants to any woman needing financial assistance for the procedure.

Still maintaining the safety record of silicone breast implants, Dow Corning Wright had suffered a "public relations disaster" ("Memos Show," 1992, p. 2A). The crisis was compared to the "classic corporate blunders" of Hooker Chemical's Love Canal, A.H. Robbins' Dalkon Shield, and Exxon's Valdez oil spill (Byrne, 1992, p. 33). Dow

Corning's reactions to the implant controversy provided us with an opportunity to extend our analysis to consider public relations strategies in health care.

When health risks are brought to public attention, the assignment of blame can be placed on physicians, government agencies, patients, manufacturers, or ambiguous agents like "society." In the scramble to sort out the safety of silicone implants, charges of negligence were leveled against various parties by different people. Our interviews revealed that some doctors blamed patients with psychological problems, sick women blamed plastic surgeons, and plastic surgeons and satisfied women with implants blamed the media for sensationalizing the risks. Although chapter 7 demonstrated the media's scapegoating of plastic surgeons, manufacturers also received a significant amount of blame, especially in television news.

Although Dow Corning was not the only implant manufacturer involved in the debate, it bore the brunt of criticisms and accusations of unethical practices regarding breast implant production and research. Media reports focused primarily on Dow Corning's role in the development, manufacture, and sales of silicone implants. National television news, in particular, highlighted Dow's role, reporting on the company's actions almost 100 times between 1990 and 1992. The other manufacturers were mentioned only a few times during the same period.

The criticisms of Dow Corning placed it in a public debate, not only over implant safety, but about its corporate character as well. When Dow withdrew from the implant market, the company claimed loss of profit as its motive, but it also had lost a public battle to defend itself against charges of unethical character and action. Part of the reason for Dow's failure can be found in its press releases to the news media and the resulting media coverage. A brief history of Dow's role in the controversy provides a necessary context for our analysis of the company's press releases and corresponding media coverage.

DOW CORNING'S IMPLANT HISTORY

When Dow Corning introduced silicone breast implants in 1964, the devices were hailed as a significant improvement over the liquid silicone injections that had been used to augment women's breasts since the 1940s. Because the implants were encased in a silicone envelope, they reduced the risk of leakage and displacement, and plastic surgeons were enthusiastic about their use. As a result, Dow's new implants became commercially successful, dominating the market until 1972 when McGhan Medical Corporation began selling a fluid gel silicone implant that felt more elastic and natural than the Dow product, which was said to have a "rubbery" feel. Dow Corning responded to the competition in 1975 by forming the Mammary Task Force to direct the design, testing, manufacturing scale-up, and product introduction of . . .

1. Low Profile Round and Low Profile Contour shapes in a variety of sizes.
2. Development and introduction of a more responsive gel material.
3. Design and introduction of a new sterile package. (Dow Corning, 1992e, p. 1)

Dow introduced its new low profile implants in June 1975.

During the time Dow had been manufacturing implants, the devices had been unregulated. But, in 1976, Congress passed a law that extended the FDA's jurisdiction to include approval of the safety and effectiveness of medical devices. Since breast implants were already on the market, they were "grandfathered in" and approved retroactively on the basis of a future review.

In 1979, the FDA organized an advisory panel to review implants. During that 1982 to 1984 review, the panel found that implants could rupture and cause other complications. Based on this information, it concluded that insufficient data existed on which to approve the marketing of silicone implants. Later, in 1983, the panel voted to maintain the devices as "Class III" products, which required that manufacturers provide safety and efficacy information. The panel also recommended that the FDA give implants "the highest priority for immediate review" (Castleman, 1991, p. 105).

The FDA was not the only forum in which Dow Corning was forced to defend its implants. During the period between 1978 and 1991, Dow Corning faced numerous lawsuits seeking damages for alleged implant malfunctions (Castleman, 1991). Most were settled successfully by Dow. Two suits, however, changed the allegations from damages for implant malfunctions to charges of unethical and fraudulent actions: *Stern v. Dow Corning* and *Hopkins v. Dow Corning*.

In 1983, Maria Stern filed suit against Dow Corning, claiming her ruptured silicone gel breast implants were the cause of her autoimmune disease (*Stern v. Dow Corning*). Prior to this filing, Dow Corning had "settled dozens of similar cases for small amounts" (Castleman, 1991, p. 48). However, on examination of Dow Corning archives, Stern's lawyers discovered internal documents that suggested the company had prior knowledge of high rupture risk and inflammatory reactions that could result from ruptures, inducing autoimmune diseases like Stern's. The lawyers' search also uncovered the now infamous 1971 "dog study" in which implant experiments on dogs ended with the death of one and the development of serious inflammation symptoms in three others.

In 1984, after hearing damaging testimony from toxicologists, immunologists, and surgeons, and learning about Dow's internal documents, the jury awarded Stern $211,000 in compensatory damages and $1.5 million in punitive damages. Dow appealed the verdict, but before the appeal could go to trial, the parties reached a settlement. Part of this resolution was to seal the documents associated with the trial. A year later, Dow Corning included product inserts in implant packages to warn women and doctors of possible complications associated with scar tissue and inflammatory reactions to silicone leakage from the rupture of silicone gel implants. Physicians were instructed to give the information to their patients (Hilts, 1992a; Smart, 1991).

Meanwhile, in 1988, after taking a "bureaucratic hiatus," the FDA notified manufacturers that they would need to seek Pre-Market Approvals (PMAs) proving the safety of their products (Castleman, 1991). However, before Dow Corning submitted its safety data, a public controversy erupted challenging its ability to continue marketing silicone gel implants and to maintain its credible corporate image.

In December 1990, *Face to Face with Connie Chung* aired a story about women who were seriously ill, claiming that silicone breast implants were to blame (Lack, 1990). Although physicians, plastic surgeons, and manufacturers maintain that the program was full of misinformation, the show triggered a national conflict among women patients, plastic surgeons, the FDA, and implant manufacturers. In our interviews with women who had health problems, the program was mentioned as alerting women to potential problems and leading some to diagnose themselves with implant- related illnesses. Plastic surgeons told us that *Face to Face* generated large numbers of phone calls and visits from concerned patients, most of whom had no symptoms, but were worried by the information in the program.

In the midst of growing media attention and public concern, Dow filed PMA safety information by the required April 1991 date. But, 5 months later, the FDA required further scientific data from Dow Corning and three other breast implant manufacturers in order to complete their safety review because of "deficiencies in their pre-market approval applications" (Dow Corning, 1992g, p. 2).

During this time, the FDA itself came under increasing criticism. The Command Trust Network, Congressman Ted Weiss, and national television news reports accused the agency of not doing enough to ensure implant safety and patient protection. In November 1991, pressured by media reports, consumer advocacy groups, and research information suggesting a link between the polyurethane foam also used to coat some breast implants and cancer in animals, the FDA called a special Advisory Committee meeting to determine the safety of breast implants and to recommend whether they should remain on the market. The committee requested more research, not a ban on silicone implants; but the controversy would not wait for additional studies. In February the committee was to be assembled again. Also in November 1991, the *Face to Face with Connie Chung* program on implants was rebroadcast, increasing public concern (Lack, 1990).

Throughout the dispute, Dow steadfastly affirmed the safety and efficacy of its product. The company continuously reiterated the benefits of the implant to millions of women, and sharply criticized the media for sensationalizing a few stories and minor problems. Dow cited years of scientific research that proved the implants were not a health risk. And then a bomb dropped.

In June 1991, Mariann Hopkins' liability suit against Dow Corning was scheduled to go to trial. The case claimed that the company had previous knowledge of health dangers related to silicone gel (*Hopkins v. Dow Corning*). Hopkins had been diagnosed with mixed connective tissue disease in 1979 after her implants ruptured, spilling silicone into her chest. Her lawyers successfully petitioned to use the documents from the Stern case and found additional damaging documents at the

Dow Corning headquarters. These included a 1974 study that showed silicone to be an "immunostimulant—a substance that provokes the type of immune reaction that goes awry in autoimmune disease" (Castelman, 1991, p. 105). In December 1991, Hopkins was awarded $7.3 million in punitive damages. The jury ruled that Dow Corning did have previous knowledge and was therefore partially responsible for misinformation leading to damages. The national media gave prominent coverage to the verdict and to the existence of Dow's damaging internal documents.

Under heavy media pressure, Dow agreed to disclose the internal memos and documents, used in both cases and sealed by the courts, to the press. The documents were presented by critics and the media as evidence that Dow knew about health and aesthetic problems associated with silicone gel implants. The company was accused of unethical behavior as national news media printed and broadcast excerpts from internal memos by Dow scientists and marketing representatives expressing concerns that silicone gel could cause serious immune system health problems.

The controversy erupted as members of the American Association of Plastic and Reconstructive Surgeons, Dow Corning, the Public Citizen's Health Research Group, rheumatologists, scientists, lawyers, politicians, and women with implants, met in Washington in February 1992 to testify. The media coverage of the meetings fueled further accusations against Dow. The company faced a highly publicized legal, economic, and ethical crisis.

DOW DEFENDS ITSELF

Although corporate America is motivated by profit, society expects its businesses to be good citizens, as well as good capitalists. Businesses are expected to demonstrate social responsibility, especially companies we rely on to protect and promote our health. While acknowledging the corporation's primary goal of returning profit to shareholders, the public expects business to conduct its affairs ethically. It holds corporations accountable for perceived ethical violations. The recent business crises of Exxon (the Valdez) and Johnson & Johnson (Rely tampons) demonstrate how companies are scrutinized and attacked when products, services, or operations cause harm to the public.

Corporate actions in the face of such crises are taken as reflections of their policies, and their policies are seen as statements of their ethics. Thus, organizations are conferred with a moral identity. With this morality comes the importance of maintaining a socially responsible character, one that reveals a commitment to good "citizenship" (see, e.g., Dionisopoulos & Vibbert, 1983, 1988; McMillian, 1987).

Like other corporations who have been charged with fraud and/or misconduct, Dow was presented with a crisis of corporate character. The company had been accused of knowingly marketing a product that might cause illnesses and aesthetic complications in millions of women. Like other organizations, Dow relied on press releases as the primary means for communicating its defense to the public. Between

December 1991 and December 1992, at the height of media and FDA attention to the controversy, Dow Corning Wright issued 25 press releases specifically focused on silicone breast implants. We obtained these documents from the company and analyzed them. We considered the releases to be the means by which Dow attempted to present and repair its image of social responsibility and to cope with the mediated reshaping of its defense against charges of unethical behavior. These press releases present the company's strategies for confronting the attacks on its corporate character.

Dow's Defense: A Failure of Corporate Apologia

Guidelines for successful crisis management include accepting responsibility for problems associated with a company's product and disclosing all information relevant to the case (Byrne, 1992). Dow Corning's press releases did neither. Instead, its strategy was threefold: First, the company dissociated itself from the charges; second, it attempted to bolster its image; and third, it scapegoated the media (see, e.g., Dion-isopoulos & Vibbert, 1983, 1988; Hearit, 1993; Ware & Linkugel, 1973).

Dissociation Tactics

In its press releases, Dow Corning attempted to dissociate itself from accusations of wrongdoing by creating a division between science and opinion. The company characterized the silicone implant controversy as a battle between science and politics (based on opinion). Dow placed itself and its safety research in the scientific camp and relegated its opponents to the realm of innuendo, rumor, and anecdote:

> [Dow has] provided substantial scientific studies that support the safety of [breast implants] and the absence of immune system response. Unfortunately, what we have in this process [the FDA hearing] is a cloud of uncertainty based on speculation and anecdotal clinical observation, not mainstream science that stands up to peer review among experts. (Dow Corning, 1992b)

These dissociation tactics were Dow's dominant public response. They: (a) reinforced the scientific process used by Dow, (b) characterized implant risks as known and accepted scientific knowledge, and (c) denied that Dow's actions and problems were caused by lack of scientific rigor or certainty.

Dow characterized its implant design and development as the result of a comprehensive scientific process. Any action to restrict implants was portrayed as lacking rigor. When the FDA called for a voluntary moratorium of silicone gel breast implants on January 6, 1992, Dow Corning complied with the request, but protested, urging the FDA to "bring science back into this decision" (Dow Corning, 1992b). For Dow, scientific process meant long-term studies, comprehensive research, and scientific testimony. The company's press releases claimed that years of scientific research and experience had proven the safety of its silicone implants (Dow Corning, 1992b). Dow claimed the scientific criteria of long-term studies and multiple tests for its own research: "In fact we believe that Dow Corning's accumulated safety studies on silicone implants is the most comprehensive body of knowledge amassed for an implantable device" (Dow Corning, 1992d).

Asking for the FDA to join Dow in the appropriate scientific process, the manufacturer claimed "if this review is done with experts in immunology, we're confident the process will support the safety of breast implants" (Dow Corning, 1992b). Almost 80% of the releases focused on the importance of examining questions about implants from a scientific perspective.

Even when Dow took actions and made statements that recognized problems associated with the devices, the manufacturer relied on the science-opinion split. When media reports linked implants to a large number of health complications, Dow acknowledged only minor risks, maintaining its stance on safety: "Safe does not mean risk free. But the risks are known and understood" (Dow Corning, 1992d). When Dow's incriminating internal documents were linked to the Hopkins verdict, Dow announced on January 22 that it would release all information. The press releases asked that the documents be seen in the context of a comprehensive scientific program: "The memos do not record the existing body of knowledge Dow Corning had already accumulated on the safety of silicones in the body. By 1975, we already had a foundation of safety studies on silicones in the human body dating back to the 1950s" (Dow Corning, 1992d).

Two months later, when FDA restrictions severely cut its implant market, Dow announced its decision not to resume sales of breast implants. In a press release, however, Dow maintained that the withdrawal was "not related to issues of science or safety but to the existing condition of the marketplace" (Dow Corning, 1992f). Throughout 1992, Dow Corning reiterated its history of scientific studies and safety. Over 60% of the press releases during 1992 reiterated the safety of silicone breast implants.

Bolstering

Dow's second defense strategy associated the company with something the audience valued: women's health and well-being. Dow characterized its research, development, and marketing of silicone breast implants as motivated by a concern for women. In his January 10, 1992, speech to the National Press Club, Robert T. Rylee explained the company's original purpose for developing and marketing breast implants: "We originally got into this business in the early 1960s because [a doctor] approached us to see if there wasn't something we could do to help the millions of women who faced the tragedy of breast cancer. . . . to provide women with the promise of breast reconstruction following mastectomy . . ." (Dow Corning, 1992c).

Dow's bolstering often focused on breast cancer survivors "who have faced the ravages of breast cancer" as the beneficiaries of its dedicated work (Dow Corning, 1992a). Dow characterized its actions as having sacrificed profit in order to serve the well-being of these women:

We haven't made any money in this business in the last five years. And there were many times during those years when we asked ourselves "do we really want to stay in this business?" Each time we said "we must" because thousands of doctors and millions of women were counting on us. (Dow Corning, 1992c)

As it bolstered its own image as women's benefactor, Dow portrayed the critics of silicone breast implants as harming women. The company argued that restrictions on breast implants "should be decided on science rather than on baseless innuendo and 11th hour shadowboxing. If not, the victims will be the two million American women who have implants and the thousands more who want them each year" (Dow Corning, 1992a). The press releases portrayed Dow's concern for women, and described women as the victims of Dow's opponents. Fully half of the 1992 press releases focused on the benefits of silicone breast implants for augmentation and mastectomy patients.

Scapegoating

As Dow dissociated itself from charges of unethical behavior and bolstered its image, it also engaged in scapegoating. Surprisingly, neither scientists, political critics, nor the FDA were blamed for the problems associated with the controversy. Instead, the media became Dow's target. Dow Corning argued continuously that the media were responsible for disseminating unscientific information about the safety of implants. It rarely directly attacked the scientists and physicians that the media cited as the actual critics of the implants; nor did the company explain why its scientific studies were better than those cited by its critics. Instead, as revealed in the press releases, Dow chose to condemn the media for its role in the controversy, a "kill the messenger" strategy.

A prevalent theme in many of the Dow press releases is the politicization and sensationalism of the breast implant issue by the mass media. In about one third of the press releases Dow charged the media with alarming and confusing women with "speculation" and "sensationalist coverage." In its release criticizing the jury award to Hopkins, Dan Hayes, President and Chief Executive Officer of Dow Corning Wright said:

It's no wonder a jury can ignore the science when some media serve up sensational tabloid journalism like the Connie Chung show, and re-hash the same one-side, inflammatory claims about breast implants made by Phil Donahue. . . . Not only is it difficult for a jury to make a decision, but it is virtually impossible for women to make an informed choice about breast implants, when the inaccurate and sensational side of this story so dominates the media. (Dow Corning, 1991)

In Dow's January 13, 1992 release affirming the safety of implants, the company chastised the media for publicizing a 15-year-old memo in which a company employee recalled "crossing his fingers" while discussing the safety and efficacy of the company's implants with plastic surgeons. The media interpreted this act as a sign of dishonesty, rather than as hopefulness or promise. The Dow press release claims, "this is probably one of the best examples . . . of how a single memo taken out of context can distort reality. The result is a relentless disruption to the scientific review of breast implants" (Dow Corning, 1992d). Dow contended that, if the media would suspend references to unproven, unscientific innuendos, then the FDA would be able to fully review Dow's premarket approval application and ease the concerns of women throughout the country. Dow attempted to draw a distinction between media coverage (the memos and criticisms) and its own statements of scientific safety of implants, thus characterizing the media as detractors from knowledge. Rather than discrediting the specific critics or studies that challenged safety claims, Dow indicted the media for covering the "unfounded" charges. The company scapegoated the media as the instigator of the debate and the cause for unnecessary alarm that resulted in harm to women.

MEDIA RESPONSES

Dow's press releases attempted to vindicate the company's character by providing media sources with a science-versus-opinion frame through which to view the controversy. The company hoped to bolster its image through association with rigorous research and goodwill toward women, particularly mastectomy patients. How did the media reports about Dow Corning and its safety record correspond to Dow's dissociation, bolstering, and scapegoating? The media accounts challenged Dow's characterization of implant critics as nonscientists. The news accounts provided criticism of Dow's research program, individual studies, and claims to comprehensive knowledge. Finally, reports challenged Dow's image of goodwill.

Media Feature Criticism From the Scientific Community

Although Dow's releases attempted to draw a distinction between science (Dow) and opinion (Dow's critics), newspaper, magazine, and television news stories erased the division between Dow and its critics by placing Dow's opponents within the science community. The media included criticism about implant safety and Dow Corning's research from credible scientists, physicians, and plastic surgeons. Most damaging were safety questions from Dow's own scientists.

As Dow issued press releases claiming the safety of breast implants, the media offered opposing viewpoints from reliable scientific sources. In its report on the FDA Advisory Committee meeting, the *New York Times* cited a number of scientists and physicians who claimed complications and/or illnesses might result from implants. According to the article:

The researchers all said that a link between silicone and auto-immune disease had not been established. But they said there is a strong suspicion that silicone can cause an auto-immune disease similar yet distinct from the standard arthritis-like diseases. . . . Further, one physician from Baylor University reported that he has seen seven implant recipients with amyotrophic lateral sclerosis, a degenerative neurological condition. . . . Because the disease is rare, the high number of cases in one doctor's practice suggests a link, said Dr. Bernard Patten, a neurologist at Baylor. (Hilts, 1992b, p. A12)

Other articles cited research by Dr. Pierre Blais, a Canadian chemist investigating the safety of silicone gel implants, who claimed that "plastic surgeons have been putting in a lot of junk that has been very poorly manufactured. . . . I'm very fearful that the health problems we are seeing today are merely a hint of the disaster to come" (Regush, 1992, p. 29).

Physicians from a variety of specialties also challenged Dow's claims to have completed comprehensive safety research and to understand the risks associated with implants. For example, when Dow Corning issued its January press release stressing the company's support of the safety of its implants, the press followed with questions from Dr. David Kessler, the FDA commissioner:

We still do not know how often women with the implants suffer adverse effects. For example, there are reports that painful hardening of the implant can occur in anywhere from 10% to 70% of patients. We still do not know to what extent the implants interfere with mammography examinations. We still do not know whether the implants can increase a woman's risk of developing cancer. And we still do not know enough about the relationship between these devices and autoimmune and connective tissue diseases. ("FDA: Hold off," 1992, p. 1A)

Kessler's line of questions denied Dow's claims about what the manufacturer did know.

Other physicians made more damaging links between the implants and risk of disease. One NBC lead story focused on radiologists who claimed that breast implants could impede early detection of breast cancer because implants can shadow cancerous tissue (Gould & Zucker, 1991). CBS quoted rheumatologists who testified that, "based on some of the patients they've treated, they believe that silicone gel breast implants may be linked to autoimmune disease" (Sorenson, 1992b).

Even some plastic surgeons were included in news reports as sources of evidence against the implant's safety and efficacy. The media coverage of Dow's internal documents in February 1992, revealed numerous complaints from plastic surgeons about the company's product. A *St. Petersburg Times* article highlighted these doctors' criticisms:

Included in the book were nearly 20 pages of computer printouts simply listing the complaints the company has received on the implants. Most involved rupture of the implant, but there were also reports of leakage (gel bleed), discoloration, bubbles, sterilization, infection, optical nerve atrophy and tumors. In one complaint, a doctor in Las Vegas said in a 1987 letter he felt "like a broken record" making his complaints. ("Memos Show," 1992, p. 2A)

Media accounts of criticism and complaints from Dow's own scientists and customers were some of the most compelling pieces of evidence undermining perceptions of implant safety. CBS reported that for years:

> [Dow Corning] ignored concerns raised by its own scientists and hid damaging information from the FDA. . . . One scientist says he resigned in protest because of insufficient data on silicone's long-term effects on body tissue. [He said] "I felt it was morally wrong and ethically wrong to implant a fluid device in the body that could release silicone fluid . . . gel." (Sorensen, 1992a)

Other Dow researchers echoed concerns over the company's lack of safety data and inadequate long-term research efforts. Following Dow's January 13 statement insisting on the safety of silicone gel implants, the *New York Times* cited a memo from ex-Dow Corning employee A. H. Rathjen, once chairman of the task force working on the silicone gel implant:

> We are engulfed in unqualified speculation. . . . Nothing to date is truly quantitative. Is there something in the implant that migrates out or off the mammary prosthesis? Yes or no! Does it continue for the life of the implant or is it limited or controlled for a period of time? What is it? (Hilts, 1992a, p. A1)

Another Dow scientist quoted in the *St. Petersburg Times* characterized Dow's investigation as inadequate:

> In one 1985 memo, Bill Boley, a company scientist, warned more testing was needed to determine whether a particular formula of the silicone gel caused cancer. He wrote, "Without this testing, I think we have excessive personal and corporate liability exposure." ("Memos Show," 1992, p. 2A)

Criticisms from Dow's own scientists and customers were widely featured in television news reports on all three major networks. ABC, CBS, and NBC literally lifted sentences from Dow's internal documents and used them as visual evidence in their coverage. Dow continued to reiterate that these documents were not accurate or representative evidence of the safety of implants, but "record only one side of an internal dialogue" (Dow Corning, 1992d). Nonetheless, the documents became standard evidence in the debate.

Criticism of Dow's Research Program

Media accounts refuted the characterization of implant critics as nonscientists. Having established that many of Dow's detractors were scientists, physicians, and plastic surgeons, the media drew the debate as a controversy within the scientific community, not, as Dow had characterized the clash, as between science and opinion. Having established the right of the critics to engage in scientific debate, the media also printed the opponents' specific attacks on Dow's research program. The critiques usually characterized the manufacturer's safety research as inadequate and failing to fulfill accepted procedures.

When commenting on Dow's 30-year record of breast cancer research, critics labeled it "inadequate" (Friedman, 1992), and characterized it as "Swiss cheese research" (Goodman, 1992, p. 16A). Of particular concern was the lack of long-term follow-up research to track women over time. After the Hopkins suit, *Newsweek* quoted a Dow scientist's memo, "To my knowledge, we have no valid long-term implant data to substantiate the safety of gel for long-term implant use" (Seligmann, Cowley, & Springer, 1992, p. 45). NBC reported that a Dow scientist complained that, "We have no valid long-term implant data to substantiate . . . safety." (Gould & Zucker, 1992a). Another *Newsweek* article reported that 7 years after initial requests from Dow scientists to "begin in-depth study" of implant ruptures, another company scientist "was still warning that 'we have no valid long-term data to substantiate the safety of gels for long-term implant use'" (Cowley et al., 1992, p. 56).

Critics also accused Dow of failing to follow accepted procedures for the research, development, and marketing of medical devices and drugs. The *St. Petersburg Times* reported a Congressional investigation on "evidence that Dow Corning Corp. may have broken federal laws in selling its silicone gel breast implants" ("Lawmaker," 1992, p. 7A). The report quoted the chair of the House subcommittee that oversees the FDA, "the company may have misbranded the device, withheld relevant safety information, failed to report serious risks associated with the device and or misrepresented their safety data" ("Lawmaker," 1992, p. 7A).

The media printed numerous accusations that Dow failed to report or follow-up on the negative results of research studies. Following the release of Dow's internal documents, *Business Week* stated that the documents "may show that the company misrepresented its safety data on implants for more than 15 years" (Galen, Byrne, Smart, & Woodruff, 1992, p. 36). A study in which implants were placed in dogs was often referenced by Dow's critics:

> [During the FDA Advisory Committee meeting] Rep. Ted Weiss of New York wrote Kessler a letter saying that [Dow] may have suppressed damaging research results. He alluded to a 1970 implant study involving several dogs. The animals developed harmless tissue responses to the implants after six months. More severe inflammations developed after two years. But instead of reporting that development and tracking it, Dow Corning put the dogs to death and later published an article describing their condition as unchanged. (Cowley et al., 1992, p. 56)

ABC quoted FDA Advisory Panel member Dr. Norman Anderson, who called the dog experiments "a peculiar phenomenon . . . which must be unprecedented in the history of device regulation" (Friedman, 1992).

The dog study was the most frequently cited experiment that critics said Dow misrepresented. However, it was not the only example. A research project on autoimmune reactions also came back to haunt the manufacturer. Throughout the controversy, Dow asserted that no scientific research had linked silicone to autoimmune problems. During the 1992 FDA hearings, a study conducted by a Dow scientist in 1974 was discussed. The experiment on guinea pigs found a link between silicone and immune system responses, "One of Dow Corning's top scientists discovered in 1974 that silicones—including some forms in breast implants—can trigger powerful reactions by the immune system" ("74 Study," 1992, p. 6A). When the scientist in charge of the study was asked about the experiment during the 1992 FDA hearings, he denied the early conclusion, "that was not much of an experiment. . . . we were just fooling around" ("74 Study," 1992, p. 6A). A *St. Petersburg Times* article characterized the study as much more than "fooling around," reporting that the conclusions of the research were signed and approved by the researchers, asking for continued follow-up ("74 Study," 1992, p. 6A).

Other reports criticized Dow's research procedures and process. According to *U.S. News and World Report*, "a doctor reviewing 10,000 pages of Dow Corning records for the FDA has asserted that in numerous animal studies, implants were not placed in or under breast tissue, an error he called 'unprecedented in the history of medical-device evaluation'" ("Breast Implants," 1992, p. 17). The media also printed criticism that Dow had failed to complete animal studies prior to using the implants on women, "The company implanted devices in women even before collecting scientific data from animal studies" (Sorenson, 1992a). According to a *New York Times* article, internal memos and documents included:

> A report dated Feb. 7, 1975, describes studies on rabbits showing "mild to occasionally moderate acute inflammatory reaction" that might be explained by the surgery itself on the rabbits, rather than by silicone leaks. But even before these results were in, eight women in Canada had received the new implants in what the company described as a "clinical experiment." (Hilts, 1992a, p. B10)

The implantation of these devices in women before long-term studies were complete led critics to label the use of silicone implants as human experimentation:

> Only now, after decades of breast implants, are we learning that women were part of some vast experiment. Perhaps "experiment" is too scientific a word for the poorly researched and weakly regulated free market in silicone. . . . But most stunning is the discovery of just how little research was done over three decades. (Goodman, 1992, p. 16A)

Newsweek provided visual commentary in a cartoon in which a Dow Corning representative tells a group of shocked and angry-looking women, "We're testing breast implants on you, to see if they're safe for guinea pigs" (Cartoon, 1992, p. 15).

Although the media printed Dow's claims that its research supported the safety of silicone implants, news reports included many more references to critics' statements about the lack of comprehensive, appropriate, long-term research. The reports supported a label that was used frequently in 1992, that the implants were "untested." Janice Buck, a woman who believed she suffered from silicone disease, was dismayed, "I thought everything was approved by the FDA. I never dreamed there were things out there that hadn't been tested" (Mason, 1992, p. 1D). A member of the FDA advisory panel, a physician from Temple University, came to the same conclusion following the committee's review of testimony and related documents, "We simply cannot continue to implant an inadequately tested device in women" (Gould & Zucker, 1992b).

Thus, the media coverage of the controversy refuted Dow's characterization of itself as the only source of scientific and reliable information on breast implants and its critics as anecdotal charlatans. Dow's detractors were represented in the media as credible scientists, researchers, and physicians, who based their claims about implant safety on careful review of Dow's research methods. The impact of their arguments was often strengthened by the use of supporting evidence from Dow's internal memos and documents.

The Media Undermine Dow's Image as a Benefactor to Women

At the same time that Dow Corning press releases attempted to portray the company as a corporate citizen with an historic concern for women and their welfare, media accounts undermined this image of goodwill. News reports included characterizations of the company as driven by profit, dishonest to women, and concerned only with legal protection.

CBS illustrated public perception of Dow as profit oriented. A woman with implants said she was duped by Dow. "It's criminal . . . that they would allow this to go on in order to enhance their pocketbooks. There was no regard for the value of our life" (Sorenson, 1992a). A week later, Columnist Anna Quindlen echoed the characterization of Dow Corning's business orientation. She labeled the controversy over implants as "business as usual" for Dow Corning "a company that manufactures silicone implants and has sold millions of them. . . . [whose] primary concern was sales, not safety" (Quindlen, 1992, p. 8A).

Media reports confounded Dow's efforts to bolster its image by printing accusations that the company lied to women. When Dow installed an information call-in number for women concerned about implant safety, the media ran reports that the hot line misrepresented its safety information. According to a *Times* story:

> [The company was accused by the FDA] of giving out misleading information about breast implants on its hot line. . . . "[The Hotline operators] overstate the safety of breast implants and minimize known or suspected side effects," said the letter from Ronald M. Johnson, a compliance director for the agency. . . . The agency said operators had told callers that the silicone implants were "100 percent safe" and that "there have never been health problems with implants or silicone." Mr. Grupp said it was "inconceivable to me how anybody at Dow Corning would say that implants are 100 percent safe." ("After U.S. Warning," 1992, p. 8A)

ABC quoted FDA officials who called the hot line advice "false, confusing, or misleading" (Friedman, 1991). When Dow attempted to repair its relationship with women patients by offering financial support to those who wished to remove their breast implants, the company was portrayed as stingy and self-interested. A *St. Petersburg Times* article reported:

> [Dow] would contribute up to $1,200 per patient, based on financial need, for any woman to have her implants removed if her doctor deems it necessary. But Aaron Levine, a lawyer representing women suing implant manufacturers, said it often costs more than $9,000 to remove the implants. ("Firm to Pay," 1992, p. 2A)

In a similar indictment against the company, an NBC news story included criticism of the requirement that women accepting Dow's financial assistance for removal sign away their legal rights to sue the company. The story quoted Ted Weiss who "warned there should be no strings attached. Dow Corning . . . is making an offer to pay for taking out the implant in return for a waiver of legal rights these women may have against the company. That's outrageous" (Gould & Zucker, 1992c).

Rather than portraying Dow as a benefactor to women, the media ran reports that characterized the company as self-interested, profit oriented, litigious, and dishonest. A *St. Petersburg Times* article summed up the characterization with comments by Sidney Wolfe, director of the Public Citizen's Health Research Group, who said, "Dow's decision [to finance additional safety research studies] may mark 'the beginning of the end of one of the worst examples of commercial exploitation of women as sex objects by both the companies making the breast implants and the plastic surgeons putting them in'" ("Firm to Pay," 1992, p. 2A). The media provided an alternate vision of Dow as a company that used, rather than helped, its women customers.

IMPLICATIONS AND CONCLUSIONS

The media presented two competing truths about silicone gel implants: Dow's story about 30 years of comprehensive safety research versus its detractors' critiques of inadequacy, misrepresentation, and procedural violations. The public was faced with the responsibility of choosing what interpretation of knowledge it believed. This type of debate over scientific interpretation has been dubbed the *Gibson Law* (McCue, 1993). The Gibson Law states that, for every scientific study that one side of a debate produces, the other side produces an opposing one to refute it. In the case of the silicone breast implant, Dow's studies were refuted through critiques of its research and compounded by the sick women's horror stories, and the vilification of plastic surgeons.

When science contradicts itself, the public is ultimately responsible for choosing what they believe is the truth. Their choice is based on the perceived believability of each side of the debate. The difficulty with Dow's strategy to separate the allegations (opinion) from its scientific studies is that the audience had no reason to doubt the scientific credibility of the researchers, physicians, and FDA consultants, who were so often cited as the critics of silicone implants. Dow's press releases failed to engage in a debate with them by describing the company's studies in any detail or providing explanations to rebut their critics' charges evaluating specific studies. Nor did Dow specifically rebut conclusions based on clinical experience and women's personal stories.

Dow's most direct response to critics, as communicated through the press releases, focused on the contents of its own internal documents. The press releases maintained that company memos did not reveal its science, but were taken out of a larger research context. Yet, the research that was reported in those documents were the only specific examples of Dow's research that reached the public. Rather than offering additional examples of research that revealed implant safety, Dow dismissed the critiques as anecdotal and attacked the media. Ironically, the very scapegoat that Dow blamed for causing the controversy was the court of public information where the press releases would compete for space and attention. Dow's dissociation strategies worked against it. The company set the criterion for how the controversy should be weighed: scientific research. Yet, having set the frame for weighing the evidence, Dow did not fulfill its own standard in the debate.

The company's dissociation, bolstering, and scapegoating public relations strategies provided the public with no greater reason to believe Dow's spokespersons than its critics. Indeed, the media characterizations attacked the very basis on which credibility is based: goodwill toward others, expertise on relevant topics, and evidence of good character. The news audience had plenty of reason to doubt that Dow had women's health as its highest priority, had conducted rigorous scientific testing, or conducted itself in a socially responsible way. Most likely, the audience would agree with the frequent conclusion printed in the news and broadcast on television that the FDA "cannot assure the safety of [breast implants] at this time" ("FDA Hold Off," 1992, p. 1A). Even such a qualified conclusion refuted Dow's position of certainty and safety.

In this culture, corporations have been held responsible for meeting community and individual standards of morality and ethics (Dionisopoulos & Vibbert, 1983). Manufacturers like Dow Corning are required to fulfill the ethic of agency, just like the plastic surgeons discussed in chapter 7. In the case of health care, the expectations are greater than for other business ventures. As Anna Quindlen concluded in her newspaper column:

> We know that unsatisfactory products are sold all the time. But finding a split seam in your new suit and having a doctor dig stray bits of silicone gel out of your chest wall are two different things. It would be grand to know that those who manufacture body parts hold themselves to a higher standard than the makers of acrylic sweaters. (Quindlen, 1992, p. 8A)

Corporations involved in public controversies about safety are essentially involved in a debate about corporate responsibility and character that warrants specific rebuttals to critics, rather than attacks on the channels through which those charges are communicated to the public. Corporate attacks on the media for revealing questions or concerns about product safety are primarily unsuccessful because the media are perceived as fulfilling their role as defined by the public. The public demands businesses to do their jobs; to act responsibly and morally within society while producing effective and safe products.

If a corporation fails in the eyes of the public, its attempts to defend itself by scapegoating an external force and/or individual may be unsuccessful, because, ultimately, the public perceives corporations as responsible for all actions associated with its business. And once a corporation has lost credibility through charges of wrongdoing, the public withdraws its trust. As a result, all of the company's communication is "filtered through layers of consumer doubt, mistrust, and cynicism" (McCue, 1993, p. 242). Charges that someone or something else is responsible for the breach in corporate morality and ethics are also sifted through public distrust and, thus, become unsubstantial.

On March 19, 1992, Dow withdrew from the silicone breast implant market, still claiming the safety of its product. Apparently, the company lost the battle for public approval, in part, due to its unsuccessful defense. Dow failed to tell the story of a company working hard to get good information and to protect consumers. The predominant media narratives in the controversy remained the horror stories of women who believed their implants had made them ill. The most dramatic narratives about Dow Corning were those of a company that ignored attempts by its own scientists to call attention to possible risks of implants, rushed the devices to market, and misrepresented its research to the government. Dow was never successful in telling a positive story about itself. The emphasis on science might have been the beginning of such a story, but the decision to blame the media and avoid refutation of its critics either through careful debate or counternarratives kept the company from becoming the character for which it had laid the foundation. Having set the standard for judgment (scientific inquiry), Dow failed to meet the requirements of science in argument (refutation, critique of science). The company did not tell its story as a careful pursuer of scientific truth for the benefit of women.

9

PUBLIC PERCEPTIONS
OF THE IMPLANT STORY

THE PROBLEM

The study of communication and silicone gel breast implants has not been a dull, dry, ivory tower research topic. It has proved the subject of lively concern everywhere we went. As we talked with friends about our research, they expressed intense interest in the issue. Some felt women had been misled by doctors and the health industry. Feminists often saw this as another example of the exploitation of women by the male medical establishment. Media critics thought the press coverage had distorted the facts. Conservatives saw a continuing decline of trust in the experts on whom we must rely to live in a complex era. Doctors lamented the traditional physician role being undermined by amateurs. Others criticized the FDA for doing too little, or too much. Some volunteered materials, often clippings from out of town papers. While the issue was being played out nationally in Congress and the FDA, it was also being pursued in conversations day after day. If people talked to us this much about implants, surely they discussed them with each other when we were not there to notice.

The more we talked to women with implants and to doctors involved in the issue and collected newspaper and magazine clippings about the implant controversy, the more curious we became about the impact all the coverage and discussion was having on the opinions of women in our community. How was this concentrated attention affecting women? They, after all, were the past and future recipients of implants.

Doctors told us that requests for implants had plummeted, so much so that some plastic surgeons were experiencing financial difficulty. One reportedly was now earning less than he paid his nurse. The percentage of women who had ever sought implants was small, however. We might reasonably have expected the implant controversy to be an issue for only a small number of women, of relatively little interest to most. Instead, the subject was all around us, the center of talk as well as political conflict. We wanted to gauge the impact of so much media attention and discussion on the public. We also wanted to supplement our interview research with a baseline against which to compare the views of women with implants.

Questions about health communication generally, such as those about perceptions of risks and benefits, about the influence of media coverage, and about the changes in the perceived role of physicians, are considered throughout this book. We wanted to see what we could learn about those questions from looking at what the public thought. The more we began to see the implant controversy as an important case study in communication about health, the more we wondered what was happening to community opinion.

METHOD

The Questionnaire

In the spring of 1992, we decided to survey women in the Tampa Bay area about their information and attitudes related to the implant question. We began by studying the written material we had assembled and by recalling key issues in our interviews. We generated the following list of questions for the study:

1. Are women in the Tampa Bay area aware of the silicone gel implant controversy?
2. What have been their primary information and opinion sources?
   a. Which sources do they use most frequently?
   b. Do the sources chosen influence their information and opinions?
3. What are their attitudes toward the silicone breast implant issue:
   a. Toward the risks of implants?
   b. Toward the benefits of implants?
   c. Toward the various characters involved:
      1) implant patients?
      2) physicians?
      3) government?
      4) science?
      5) society?
4. Does having implants affect their attitudes?
5. Does knowing someone with implants affect their attitudes?

To develop answers to these questions we designed a questionnaire containing nine information items and 23 attitude items. Twenty-one of the attitude items used a 5-point Likert scale, ranging from 5 (*strongly agree*) to 1 (*strongly disagree*). The other two attitude items asked for "yes" or "no" responses (see Fig. 9.1). Items about the risks and benefits of implants were designed to correspond to claims found frequently in both print media and interpersonal sources. Similarly, items about the characters in the controversy featured qualities ascribed to them in our interviews

1. In the last few months have you heard anything about silicone gel breast implants?   395 a. Yes   5 b. No

2. Where have you heard about them? (Circle as many as you want)
   312   a. Newspapers   119 e. Talking with friends
   374   b. Radio or TV news   42 f. Talking with a doctor
   227   c. Radio or TV talk shows   or a nurse
   193   d. Magazines   18 g. other

3.

5	4	3	2	1
strongly agree	somewhat agree	neither agree nor disagree	somewhat disagree	strongly disagree

mean

2.89   a.   Most women who have had implants will get sick from them.
2.86   b.   Most implants leak.
3.88   c.   The government has restricted the use of silicone gel breast implants.
4.07   d.   The manufacturers of implants covered up information about their danger.
2.73   e.   The danger of silicone gel implants has been exaggerated.
3.35   f.   Implants increase the chances of breast cancer.
4.06   g.   Most women who have had implants feel better about themselves.
4.68   h.   Society places too much emphasis on the size of women's breasts.
3.36   i.   Silicone gel breast implants are truly needed by women who have had their breasts removed because of cancer.
2.67   j.   Doctors have usually done a good job of explaining about possible side effects to women considering whether to have implants.
3.72   k.   The doctors who put in the implants are motivated too much by the money they make from doing it.
2.41   l.   The women who have filed lawsuits against the implant manufacturers are motivated mostly by the money they hope to receive.
3.58   m.   Implants make it harder to detect breast cancer.
2.67   n.   Women who have had implants just to look better must be willing to accept whatever happens to them.
3.04   o.   Women with implants would be smart to have them taken out.
2.85   p.   Scientists know for sure that silicone gel implants cause disease.
3.97   q.   Women who want implants should have a right to get them.
2.33   r.   Silicone breast implants are safe.
3.12   s.   Implants cause arthritis-like illness.
3.23   t.   Most implants will have to be replaced sooner or later.
1.91   u.   If I could be sure that implants were safe I would consider having them.

FIG. 9.1. Silicone gel breast implant questionnaire and results (continued on next page).

4. If someone you care about was thinking of having implants following breast removal due to cancer would you advise her to have them?
140 a. Yes   215 b. No

5. If someone you care about was thinking of having implants in order to look better (not because of cancer) would you advise her to have them?
45 a. Yes   330 b. No

6. Does someone you know have implants?
259 a. Yes   135 b. No

7. Do you have breast implants?
20 a. Yes   376 b. No

8. How old are you?
Mean = 39

9. About how much is your (or you and your spouse's) income each year?
Mean = $54,000

10. What is your occupation? _____

11. Circle what you consider to be your ethnic background.
    13   a. African American
    15   b. Hispanic
    4   c. Asian
    57   d. Native American
    297   e. Caucasian
    0   f. Pacific Islander

12. Circle the highest level of education you have had.
    2   a. Graduated from elementary school
    44   b. Graduated from high school
    133   c. Attended college
    101   d. Graduated from college
    110   e. Attended graduate or professional school

FIG. 9.1. (continued).

and in the press coverage. The questionnaire was pretested and administered in May and June 1992, near the end of the period of the most intense media coverage.

Data Analysis.   The information on the "yes-no" items generated categorical data which were analyzed first by inspection and then by using the chi-square test. Data from the Likert-type items were subjected to the appropriate Analysis of Variance (ANOVA). The Statview SE+ Graphics program performed the calculations on a Macintosh computer. Because the number of responses was often quite large, many comparisons are easy to see simply by inspection of the numbers. Indeed, in some cases, the tests of significance were really superfluous. We needed no such test, for example, to conclude that the response of "yes" by 395 out of 400 subjects to Item 1, "In the last few months have you heard anything about silicone gel breast implants?" showed an overwhelming awareness of the issue. Response data for all items are displayed in Fig. 9.1.

Subjects.   We would have liked to have drawn a random sample of all women in the Tampa Bay area, and mailed them a survey form, which all would return. Unfortunately we were not funded to be able to pay for the mailing list, let alone the postage. We faced the common need to compromise between the feasible and the ideal. Shopping mall intercepts are now done by sophisticated commercial market research groups in all the major malls in our area. The malls are no longer available to the eager University researcher with only time, not money, to spend pursuing knowledge. Our ill-fated attempt to interest flea market patrons in our survey was explained in the introduction.

We, therefore, decided that if we were to sample opinions, it would have to be from women in established groups. We identified potential groups from meeting announcements in the local papers. We called for permission and took questionnaires to the meetings. The groups who cooperated were the Business and Professional Women's Club, the Network of Executive Women, Legal Secretaries, Women in Construction, Women in Insurance, the Mothers Support Group, the Junior League, Executive Women in Sales and Marketing, the Association of Business Women, The Midday Professional Women's Club, and the Jewish Federation. To bring the total number of respondents to 400, a final group of subjects were students from a communication class at a local community college.

Although the women in these groups have gender in common with all the women in our community, they are less representative in other ways. They have both more education and income than the typical woman. Fifty-three percent of the respondents completed college, and more than half of those attended graduate or professional school. Only 12% stopped their education with high school.

The income of subjects and their spouses appears to be above average at $54,000, with a range from $4,000 to $250,000. We say "appears" because 30% left the item blank. A number of those put comments in the margins questioning why we needed this information. Many were reluctant and unwilling to tell us their incomes. Were their incomes higher or lower than those who replied? We cannot know. But we have less confidence in the income figures than in those for education. Still the two usually correlate highly. The women in our survey are surely more educated and wealthier than a randomly drawn sample would have been.

This may not be a serious drawback. The doctors we talked to about implants told us that their patients were mostly above average in income. Some younger working women with modest salaries saved for implants the way they might for a car or a vacation, but most had to be affluent to pay for an expensive procedure not covered by insurance. The 18 women who said on this questionnaire that they have breast implants and who also reported an income, have an average income of $72,000 contrasted to an average of $53,000 for those without implants. Further, our questionnaire asked for the income of "you and your spouse." Responses would necessarily be higher than if we had asked for personal income. Nonetheless, the average for our respondents is more than double the average family income in our community.

Subjects' ages ranged from 18 to 86 with an average of 39 and a standard deviation of 11.8 years. Seventy-seven percent of the sample marked Caucasian on the questionnaire. Three percent indicated African American and 4% Hispanic. One percent marked Asian and none Pacific Islander. Fifteen percent marked Native American, but a number of these had marked, then crossed out Caucasian. Others who marked Native American wrote marginal notes such as "I was born in the U.S." The percent for Native Americans is disproportional to our expectations. These marginal comments and cross outs on the questionnaires led us to believe that the term "Native American," though politically correct, confused a number of our respondents. We, therefore, disregarded that ethnic category in our analysis.

Question 6 asked whether our subjects knew someone who had implants. Two hundred and fifty-nine said "yes" and 135 said "no." The demographic differences between those who said "yes" and those who said "no" were minor. What is interesting is the fact that 66% of these women knew another woman who had implants. Implants would not seem to be a very well kept secret.

Question 7 asked our respondents if they themselves had breast implants. Twenty said "yes" and 376 said "no." As mentioned earlier the "yes" group had significantly higher incomes than the "no" group. They also differed in education. The "yes" group had fewer elementary school graduates and more graduate school attendees than the "no" respondents.

The subjects we surveyed were more educated and affluent than the averages for our community. Our respondents were also more likely to have implants. The number of American women with implants would more than double if the 5% figure of women represented in our study were applied nationwide. If women likely to choose implants are, like those surveyed, richer and more educated than the average, then our sample may be a useful one for understanding the responses of potential implant recipients. When we asked, "If I could be sure that implants were safe I would consider having them," 22% of those responding marked "agree" or "strongly agree" (Item 3u). This percentage adds further evidence that the women we surveyed are more representative of potential recipients than a random sample would be. If 22% of adult American women had implants, their number would be 21 million rather than 1 to 2 million.

RESULTS AND DISCUSSION

Knowledge of the Issue and Sources of Information

Our first research question asked if women in our area knew about the silicone gel breast implant controversy. The results are resoundingly "yes." Only 5 of 400 respondents, slightly more than 1%, had not heard about the issue in the preceding months (see Fig. 9.1).

Our second question, "Where did women hear about the issue," also helps us answer the first question. What were the most frequent sources? Because any respondent could mark as many as all of the source options, the total of number of responses far exceeded the number of respondents. A total of 1,365 source choices were made by the respondents; more than three each. Newspapers were a source for 79% of our sample, news broadcasts for 94%, talk shows for 57%, magazines for 48%, conversations with friends for 50%, conversations with doctors or nurses for 11%, and other for 5%. Other sources listed by more than one respondent were family members, attorneys, and billboards. Clearly more than one source was used by most of those surveyed. They did not rely on only a single source of information. Both print and broadcast media were used by most, and half had talked about the topic with friends. There seems little doubt, that during the first 6 months of 1992, the silicone breast implant issue was of great interest to women in the Tampa Bay area. They knew about it, they remembered the media coverage about it, and they talked about it with their friends.

There may be several reasons for this great interest. First, the topic taps into the importance of personal appearance for women, particularly as appearance connects to sexual attractiveness. Our interviews with women with implants showed their concern with whether their appearance was acceptable to others. Their own self-esteem was connected to how they looked. The survey results reinforce this concern about breasts and appearance. When we examine the results on the attitude items, we notice that the highest level of agreement was with the statement: "Society places too much emphasis on the size of women's breasts." This strong response reveals respondents' perceptions that their appearance, particularly the size of their breasts, matters, indeed, matters too much. Further, the response that "most women who have had implants feel better about themselves," was third highest on the attitude items. Increased breast size is seen as increasing self-esteem.

Second, the question of the risk of a medical procedure, most often performed by men, might have generated widespread interest in the implants as a gender issue. Arguments that medicine is practiced with a masculine bias, and that medical research too often studies only men, have become common. Plastic surgery, even more than most specialties, is overwhelmingly male. It may have been easy to see the women who reported problems with their implants as victims of insensitive male physicians, especially if women's own experiences seemed similar to the reported failures of doctors to take seriously the complaints of women with implants.

Third, the sheer volume of media attention may have created the high level of awareness. If these subjects exposed themselves frequently, as their reports indicate, to print and broadcast media content, then they are likely to have heard about the issue. As the chapters on media demonstrate, this topic was covered heavily by local and national reporters. The agenda-setting function of the media may have made our respondents aware of the issue.

Of course, all three of these influences may have been present. For whatever reasons, we can say with assurance that women in the Tampa Bay area were familiar with this health issue. Whatever attitudes they held were not the result of never having heard about the question.

Information Sources: Talking to a Doctor or Nurse

We analyzed the data to see if any source seemed to especially influence responses on the attitude items. For all but one source, there were few significant effects.

The one source variable that seemed to matter was whether a respondent had talked with a doctor or nurse about the issue. Those 42 women who had such discussions with professionals differed significantly from those who had not done so on 10 of the 21 attitude items (see Table 9.1). Those who had done so were more positive about implants than those who did not. They saw implants as safer and more beneficial. Women who talked with a health professional were more likely to think that "implant danger was exaggerated," that "women with implants feel better about themselves," that "doctors do a good job of explaining about implant side effects," that "implants are safe," and that "if they were sure implants were safe they would consider having them." They were less likely to agree that "doctors who put in implants are too interested in the money they make," that "women with implants would be smart to have them removed," that "scientists know for sure that implants cause disease," that "implants cause arthritis-like illness," and "that most implants will have to be replaced."

Further, respondents who had talked with a doctor or nurse were more likely to advise women to have implants (Items 4 and 5, Table 9.2). Fifty-six percent of those who talked to a doctor or nurse would advise implants after breast removal compared to 37% of those who had not talked to a doctor or nurse. Twenty-six percent would recommend implants for augmentation compared to 11% who had not talked to a doctor or a nurse. They were also more likely to know someone with implants and to have implants themselves ($p < .01$ for each comparison using the chi-square test). Having talked to a doctor or nurse is a most influential variable in attitudes about implants.

It is important to note in interpreting these data that just because the difference between two groups is statistically significant in a particular direction, this does not necessarily mean that one group thought implants were safe and the other did not. Item 3r is illustrative. Whereas those who had talked to a doctor or nurse disagreed less strongly that "implants were safe" ($M = 2.66$) than those who had not talked to a health professional ($M = 2.29$), their mean response was still in the disagreement direction. The mean of 2.66 is well below the midpoint of 3.00 and even further below the overall average for attitude items, 3.23. Indeed on those overall means

TABLE 9.1
Attitude Item Means for the 42 Subjects
Who Talked to a Doctor or a Nurse

Item		Talked to a Doctor or Nurse	
		Yes	No
3e	The danger of silicone gel implants has been exaggerated.	3.31	2.66 ***
3g	Most women who have implants feel better about themselves.	4.43	4.03 **
3j	Doctors have usually done a good job of explaining about possible side effects.	3.00	2.64 *
3k	Doctors who put in implants are motivated too much by the money they make doing it.	3.26	3.78 ***
3o	Women who have implants would be smart to get them out.	2.39	3.11 ***
3p	Scientist know for sure that silicone gel implants cause disease.	2.37	2.91 ***
3r	Silicone breast implants are safe.	2.66	2.29 **
3s	Implants cause arthritis-like illness	2.73	3.17 ***
3t	Most implants will have to be replaced sooner or later.	2.81	3.28 ***
3u	If I could be sure that implants were safe I would consider having them.	2.72	1.82 ***

*** $p < .01$. ** $p < .02$. * $p < .05$.

TABLE 9.2
Number of Respondents Who Talked With a Doctor or Nurse
Who Would Advise Women to Have Implants

Items	Talked to a Doctor or Nurse	yes	no
4	Would advise implants postmastectomy	22 of 39	117 of 313[*]
5	Would advise implants for cosmetic reasons only	10 of 39	35 of 333[***]

[***] $p < .01.$ [*] $p < .05.$

only three item means fell below 2.66. This value is well below the semi-interquar-tile range. Hence, we know that talking with a doctor or nurse seems to lessen the degree of disagreement, but it is not accurate to say that those who did so agreed that implants are safe.

How can we account for the difference in attitudes for those who talked with a doctor or nurse? Several explanations seem reasonable. First, we can attribute the difference to media coverage. This group of respondents had more than media sources on which to rely. Although some physicians are worried about the potential danger to a small number of implant patients, most accept the position of the FDA that, absent symptoms, there is no reason for women with implants to seek their removal. The American College of Rheumatology issued a statement on February 27, 1992, quoting the FDA that there was no convincing evidence that implants cause any generalized diseases. The American Medical Association has gone further and asked the FDA to return silicone gel implants to the market while additional research is undertaken (Council on Scientific Affairs, 1993). Although some doctors disagree strongly, the majority medical opinion seems to be that silicone gel implants are not dangerous for most women. Most doctors, then, were likely to have emphasized the safety of implants in their conversations with those who talked with them.

But, if as our chapter analyzing the media coverage of the implant controversy argues, the media paid more attention to implant problems and presented dramatic narratives of those problems, then we would expect people who had no other sources to moderate that media content to be less favorable than those who were influenced by a discussion with a doctor or nurse.

Beyond the influence of the media is a second possible explanation for the impact of having a doctor or nurse as an information source. We could attribute differences to personalized rather than generalized knowledge of physicians. With physicians, just as with congressmen and others, survey research shows that attitudes toward one's own doctor are much more positive than attitudes toward doctors generally. If the known doctor is talked to and gives a more positive "spin" to implant safety and benefit, the respondent would have been likely to be influenced. The specific doctor is credible in comparison to the abstract doctor or unfamiliar doctor in the media.

Third, we could argue that those likely to have the opportunity to talk with doctors or nurses are different from other respondents because of that. They may be more closely connected to the health care professions. One respondent, for example, noted under "occupation" that she worked in a doctor's office.

In our interviews, women who attribute illness to their implants often said that their physicians had been reluctant or unwilling to talk with them about their concerns regarding their implants. Several doctors interviewed said that few women had come to them to discuss their implants. As several women pointed out, you do not go to see a plastic surgeon when you feel fatigued and your joints ache. If plastic surgeons are concerned with what women think about their own implants and what women generally believe about the issue, they would be wise to be proactive in initiating discussion with women in face-to-face settings. Women are very aware of this issue and their attitudes seem strongly related to whether they have talked to a doctor or nurse about the question.

Information Sources: Having Implants

Having implants and knowing someone with implants were not listed among the sources of information on the questionnaire, yet it seems obvious that each of these two groups has access to information of a special kind about the implant question. The women who have implants in their bodies have direct knowledge of them. They are much more favorable about implants than are the women in our sample generally.

Research question 4 asks whether having implants affected attitudes toward the controversy. Twenty of our respondents, 5% of the sample, reported that they had breast implants. This percentage exceeds substantially the percentage of women in American society with implants. Comparison of those with implants with the others in our sample yielded a substantial number of significant differences.

These comparisons are displayed in Table 9.3, where the item average scores are grouped by three categories: risk, benefit, and characters. Items grouped as risk included references to possible difficulties with implants (e.g., "most implants leak") or to potential danger to women with implants (e.g., "most women who have implants will get sick from them"). Those items grouped as benefits include positive results of having implants (e.g., "look better" and "feel better about themselves"). Those items grouped as characters explicitly mention people and roles: women, doctors, scientists, and manufacturers. On seven of the nine risk items the difference is significant. Women with implants are less likely to agree that "most women with implants will get sick from them," that "most implants leak," that "implants increase the chances of breast cancer," that "implants cause arthritis-like illness," and that "most implants will have to be replaced." They are more likely to agree that the "danger of implants has been exaggerated" and that "implants are safe." In regard to benefits, they are more likely to agree that "women with implants feel better about themselves," and less likely to agree that "women with implants would be smart to have them out." Their view of the characters shows greater belief that implants are "truly needed by women who have had their breasts removed," that "women who want implants should have a right to get them," and that "doctors have done a good job of explaining implant side effects." They agree significantly less that "doctors who do implants are too interested in money," that "manufacturers

TABLE 9.3
Means for Key Subject Groups by Categories for Attitude Items

Items	Have Implants		Know Someone With Implants	
	Yes	No	Yes	No
I. Implant Risk				
3a	1.65	2.95***	2.73	3.18***
3b	1.80	2.92***	2.71	3.15***
3e	4.05	2.66***	2.89	2.45***
3f	2.53	3.29***	3.18	3.42
3m	3.45	3.57	3.58	3.55
3o	1.60	3.12***	2.90	3.30***
3r	3.15	2.29***	2.41	2.16
3s	2.55	3.15***	3.10	3.17***
3t	2.50	3.27***	3.16	3.38***
II. Implant Benefit				
3g	4.70	4.03***	4.22	3.73***
3i	4.20	3.32***	3.47	3.13***
3o	1.60	3.12***	2.90	3.30
III. Characters				
3g (women)	4.70	4.03***	4.22	3.73***
3i	4.20	3.32***	3.47	3.13**
3l	2.65	2.40	2.48	2.28
3n	2.30	2.69***	2.70	2.60***
3o	1.60	3.12***	2.90	3.30***
3q	4.65	3.94***	4.09	3.76***
3j (doctors)	3.42	2.64***	2.75	2.54
3k	2.95	3.77***	3.72	3.74
3d (manufacturers)	3.35	4.11***	4.00	4.19
3h (society)	4.40	4.69**	4.68	4.69
3p (science)	1.79	2.92***	2.95	2.80

*** $p < .01.$ ** $p < .02$

have covered up information about implant danger," that "society places too much emphasis on the size of women's breasts," and that "scientists know for sure that implants cause disease." Women with implants are less concerned about implant risk, more convinced of their benefits, and more favorable to most of the characters in the controversy than are women generally. They are the only ones who have heard doctors explain side effects and can base their responses about doctors' explanations on experience. They agree much more that doctors have done a good job than do women who do not have implants and, thus, have not listened to a doctor's explanation.

Table 9.4 contains data on questionnaire Items 4 and 5, which asked if respondents would advise women to have implants following mastectomies (Item 4) and to improve appearance (Item 5). Eighty-five percent of the women with implants would advise implants in response to Item 4 compared to 37% of women without implants. Twenty-nine percent of those with implants would advise implants under Item 5, whereas only 2% without implants would do so. Clearly women with implants are more likely to advise others to have them.

If any women should be worried about the risks of implants, we might expect that those who have implants would be the ones, but in fact, however, they are much less concerned. They apparently like their implants, and would recommend them to others more often than other women would. Their positive perceptions mirror those of the women we interviewed with implants who do not believe they are ill. Neither those women nor the women we surveyed share the negative views about implants of the women we interviewed who believe their implants have made them ill. The surveyed women with implants are significantly more positive on item after item than are the sample of women generally. They have the most direct experience and must rely less on the indirect reports of others and of the media. They are the most positive.

TABLE 9.4
Number of Respondents Who Have or Know Someone
Who Has Implants Advising Women to Have Implants

Items	You Have Implants		You Know Someone With Implants	
	Yes	No	Yes	No
4 Would advise implants postmastectomy	17 of 20	123 of 334 ***	107 of 231	33 of 122 ***
5 Would advise for cosmetic purposes	13 of 19	32 of 355 ***	39 of 239	6 of 134 ***

*** $p < .01$.

Information Sources: Indirect Experience

If having direct experience makes a difference in attitudes, perhaps various kinds of indirect experience also make a difference. One kind of indirect experience comes from knowing someone who has implants. Women might get information about implants from friends who have them. Research question 5 asks whether women who know others with implants differ in their attitudes toward implants. Sixty-six percent of those responding to this item know someone with implants.

Table 9.3 contains a comparison of their attitudes with those who do not know someone with implants. Differences were tested for significance using the ANOVA. In regard to risks, those who know others with implants are more likely to agree that "implant danger has been exaggerated," and that "implants are safe." They are less likely to agree that most "women with implants will get sick from them," that "most implants leak," that "implants increase the chances of breast cancer," and that "most implants will have to be replaced." On the character items they agree more strongly that "women should have a right to get implants." They also agree more that "most women with implants feel better about themselves," and that "implants are truly needed" by women who have mastectomies. They disagree more that "women with implants would be smart to have them out." Their views on the other character items do not differ significantly from those women who do not know someone with implants.

Table 9.4 shows their responses to the items about advising others to get implants. Forty-six percent of those who know someone with implants would recommend implants postmastectomy compared to 27% of the others. Whereas only 16% would recommend implants to improve appearance, a mere 5% of those not knowing someone with implants would make such a recommendation. Knowing someone with implants makes one more likely to advise their use. Women who know others with implants view the safety and benefits of implants more positively, but differ little in their attitudes toward the characters in the controversy.

There seems every likelihood that if a woman knows someone who has implants, the woman has learned about the implant experience, at least to some degree, from that person. One would expect those who know someone with implants to have a better understanding of what it is like to have them than would respondents who do not know an implant recipient. If that is the case, we could consider their experience less indirect than those who do not know someone with implants. If their experience is considered more direct because they know someone with implants, and if we remember that those with the most direct experience, those with implants, have more positive attitudes about implants, we can formulate a conclusion: The more direct the experience, the more favorable women feel about implants. (Those who attribute illness to their implants are obvious exceptions.)

Those who neither have implants nor know another woman with them might have talked to friends about the topic. Such talk is another still less direct, but personal, information source. The only significant differences attributable to talking with friends were also in the direction of more positive attitudes toward implant safety and benefit. Women who talked to friends were less likely to agree that "most women with implants will get sick from them," (Item 3a, $p < .02$) and more likely to agree that they would "want implants if they were sure they were safe" (Item 3u, $p < .02$). Women who used other sources were also more likely to agree with 3u ($p < .01$), and less likely to agree that "women with implants would be smart to have their implants removed" (Item 3o, $p < .03$). Although that source variable has much smaller influence, what influence it does have moves women in a favorable direction.

Those who relied entirely on the media as information sources are the most negative about the implant issue and the people involved in it. We believe that the impact of media coverage on these womens' attitudes reflects the nature of the media content. Recall that in chapters 6, 7, and 8, we pointed out that the coverage of risk and danger was in narrative form while the coverage of safety and benefits was, for the most part, in rational form. Further, the negative depiction of the doctors and the manufacturers was in narrative form. Positive stories about the characters were virtually absent, as were narratives about implant benefits. If narrative discourse is especially persuasive, then we should expect those who relied on these media narratives to find implants more dangerous and less beneficial than those who had other sources. We would expect them to view the characters depicted negatively as more malicious. That is, indeed, what we found. It seems fair to say that the media coverage has increased the belief that implants are risky and that those involved in the controversy have not acted in the interests of patients and society. We can attribute much of that effect to the use of narratives to explain danger and personal irresponsibility, and rational discourse to explain their opposites.

ATTITUDES

Overall Attitudes

Our third research question asks what attitudes women have toward the breast implant issue. Table 9.5 lists the average scores on attitude items in rank order. Agreement that "society places too much emphasis on the size of women's breasts" (Item 3h) is the highest for any item, more than six tenths of a point higher than the next highest item. The other items with average agreement scores above four are that "manufacturers covered up information about implant danger" (3d) and that "women with implants feel better about themselves" (3g). The item least agreed with, "if I knew implants were safe I would want them," is the only one to fall below a mean of two (3u). The next lowest agreement scores are "implants are safe" (3r) and "women who are suing manufacturers are too interested in money" (3l). The average of all average agreement scores is 3.23, showing a tendency of respondents to agree somewhat more than disagree with the items. This average may reflect their strong feeling about a few items because the average score for only 9 items fell above 3.23 and 12 fell below.

We were interested in whether the women we surveyed had responded differently to statements of different kinds. We grouped the attitude items into three categories: those having to do with the risks of implants; those having to do with the benefits of implants; and those referring to the characters involved in the implant controversy: women, doctors, manufacturers, scientists, and society. In Table 9.5, each item is marked according to its category. Note that several items appear more than once. These items have more than one dimension. Inspection of the categories shows that the character items appear most often in the top and bottom ranks, whereas the risk items appear in the midranks for the most part. The three benefit

TABLE 9.5
Overall Sample Values for the Likert Items in Rank Order

Mean	Item	Category
4.68	3h	Aso
4.07	3d	Am
4.06	3g	B, Aw
3.97	3q	Aw
3.88	3c	—
3.72	3k	Ad
3.58	3m	R
3.36	3i	B, Aw
3.35	3f	R
3.23	mean of the means	
3.23	3t	R
3.12	3s	R
3.04	3o	R, B, Aw
2.89	3a	R
2.86	3b	R
2.85	3p	Asc
2.73	3e	R
2.67	3j	Ad
2.67	3n	Aw
2.41	3l	Aw
2.33	3r	R
1.91	3u	—

Category codes: R = Risk, B = Benefits, and A = characters: w = women; d = doctor; so = society; sc = scientists; m = manufacturers.

items are spaced throughout. Of the seven items that fall within the semi-interquartile range, six are risk items. The respondents have stronger beliefs about the characters in the breast implant controversy than about the risk or benefits of implants. They both agreed and disagreed more strongly on the character items.

Items 3c and 3u were not assigned to any category. The former was an information accuracy check. Because the FDA had restricted implant use, we would expect respondents to say that it had done so. The score obtained, 3.88, was fifth highest. We would expect a low score on Item 3u because only a small percentage of women get implants; estimates vary between 1 and 2 million nationally. The score obtained was the lowest at 1.91. Remember, however, that 22% of our subjects agreed or strongly agreed with Item 3u, a much higher percentage than the percentage of women who actually have implants.

Items 4 and 5 asked the respondents what advice they would give women considering having implants; Item 4 for women who had lost breasts due to cancer, and Item 5 for women who wanted to look better. Of the 355 women responding to Item 4, 140 said "yes." Of the 375 responding to Item 5, 45 said "yes." Although more than three times as many respondents would recommend implants following mastectomies than for cosmetic augmentation, fewer than 40% would recommend implants at all (see Table 9.4).

Five Patterns

The attitudes of our subjects present some interesting patterns. The first pattern can be seen in responses to the form of the attitude items. Throughout our work we have argued that narrative discourse is special. It has special power for people both as they talk about their lives, and as they process what they hear, read, and view.

Attitudes Toward Characters.   When we looked at the attitude items we found that those referring to characters taking action generated stronger responses, either agreement or disagreement, than those that contained no characters. The average scores for items with characters occupy most of the highest and lowest ranks of the 21 items. These character items, although certainly not full narratives, do contain the basic elements of a narrative. Someone does something. It is fascinating that they generate stronger reactions than the straightforward abstract propositions. This pattern provides further evidence for the idea that narrative discourse generates stronger responses than rational discourse.

Attitudes Toward Cancer.   A second pattern emerges from the items about cancer on the survey form. Women perceive a strong connection between breast implants and breast cancer. Three attitude items refer to cancer: 3f, 3i, and 3m. Their average scores are all above the overall average. We compared the scores for the cancer items to those about disease in general and about other specific illnesses. For those other items the average scores were below the overall average score. Cancer is the potential health problem to which women react most strongly.

In addition, Item 4 asked respondents whether they "would advise women to have implants after breast removal due to cancer." Thirty-nine percent said "yes," whereas only 12% would advise implants "to make a woman look better" in response to Item 5.

The connections outside of our study between breasts, implants, and cancer are powerful. Estimates suggest that up to one third of women with implants have had them after breast removal due to cancer. Such women argued before the FDA that their implants played a vital role in their psychological recovery from mastectomy. They feared that women in the future would be unwilling to undergo breast removal if implants were unavailable. The FDA accommodated their views by allowing silicone gel implants to be available postmastectomy, but not for cosmetic augmentation.

In addition to these connections between cancer and implants, we discovered in our interviews women whose fear of breast cancer is so intense that they underwent subcutaneous mastectomies prophylactically. All the breast tissue is scraped from inside the skin of the breast in the hope that any potential cancer can be eliminated before it develops. Some have the nipple removed lest breast tissue remain in it, unremoved. The anxiety that leads to the desire for this procedure is often linked to a strong family history of breast cancer, and/or the presence of fibroids in the breast. Following the operation, most of these women had implants put in. Some underwent the tram flap operation in which muscle from the abdomen is used to create a new breast. Others had no reconstruction.

These women spoke at length to us in our interviews about their vision of breast cancer as a scourge. Yet, the surgeons we talked to felt such operations were unwise and most would no longer perform them, even on request. They argued that, because research shows no advantage for this procedure in preventing cancer, the procedure offers more harm than benefit. In chapter 5, we explained that some physicians believe women with subcutaneous mastectomies differ psychologically from other patients. The women we talked to had chosen these operations, sometimes against their physicians' advice, in the desperate hope that they would not fall victim to breast cancer.

Although their views may be more extreme than those of most women, the fear of cancer and its connection with the breast extends to perceptions about implants by women generally. Much of the concern about implants was expressed as concern about the relation to cancer.

The New England Journal of Medicine carried a very reassuring article in its June 18, 1992 issue. Canadian researchers Berkel, Birdsell, and Jenkins took advantage of the fact that Alberta's health insurance plan had paid for breast augmentation and, consequently, they had access to records of a kind not available in the United States. They studied nearly 12,000 women who had breast augmentation between 1973–1986. They compared them with the more than 13,500 breast cancer cases diagnosed during that period and found that the women with implants were less likely than the general population to get breast cancer. This study was not widely reported in the popular press, however, and appeared after our survey.

Our interviews with women with implants revealed a strong fear of breast cancer. The results of our survey reinforce that concern as it is linked to silicone gel breast implants. It is probably impossible to talk about health and the breast without the concern for cancer becoming prominent.

Attitudes Toward Women With Implants.   A third pattern in the results expresses a generally positive attitude toward women who have chosen to have implants. The third highest average score on the attitude items was for 3g, "most women with implants feel better about themselves." Two items offered the opportunity to criticize women with implants: 3n, "women who have implants just to look better must be willing to accept whatever happens to them," and 3i, "the women who have filed lawsuits against implant manufacturers are motivated mostly by the money they hope to receive." Their average scores ranked 19th and 18th out of 21 respectively. In contrast, 3k, "the doctors who put in implants are motivated too much by the money they make from doing it," ranked sixth. In informal discussion, women with implants are sometimes described in pejorative terms as vain, shallow, and self-obsessed, but that view was not reflected in the results of our survey. Despite the fact that only one in eight of our respondents would advise someone they cared about to have implants just to look better, they were not critical, and overwhelmingly supported the belief that women who want implants have a right to get them.

Attitudes Toward Responsible Parties.   The fourth pattern reflected in these results is the critical attitude toward those who were supposed to be responsible for making sure implants were safe. These characters were viewed negatively:

1. Society places too much emphasis on the size of women's breasts. (Ranked 1st)
2. Manufacturers of implants covered up information about their danger. (Ranked 2nd)
3. Doctors
    a. who put in implants are motivated too much by the money they make doing it. (Ranked 6th)
    b. have usually done a good job of explaining about possible side effects to women considering whether to have implants. (Ranked 17th)

The overwhelming support for a woman's right to choose implants (Ranked 4th) flies directly in the face of the ruling by the FDA restricting access, issued April 16, 1992, the month before our survey was begun. That result also shows criticism of those in charge, particularly when we notice that our respondents knew that implant use had been restricted, "the government has restricted the use of silicone gel breast implants" (ranked 5th). Our respondents knew they were restricted, but nonetheless affirmed a woman's right to choose implants. Across a series of items, the women we surveyed placed much blame on those responsible for health care safety.

Attitudes Toward Implant Safety.   The final pattern of responses shows a level of caution by respondents about the safety of implants. Most respondents disagreed with safety items regardless of their positive or negative orientation. Ranked in the bottom 10 are statements that "implants are safe," and that "the danger has been exaggerated." Results also indicate disagreement with Items 3o, that "women would be smart to have implants out," 3a, "that most women will get sick from their implants," and 3b, that "most implants leak." The best explanation of this pattern may be the respondents' disagreement with Item 3p, that "scientists know for sure that silicone gel implants cause disease" (ranked 15th). In the face of this uncertainty, the women we surveyed disagreed with statements that said implants were safe and that implants were unsafe. We believe this pattern suggests good judgment on an important health issue about which considerable uncertainty existed at the time of the controversy.

Demographic Differences

Only a few of the statistical tests run on the variables of age, income, and education yielded significant differences. None of the findings suggested useful patterns. Readers who wish to see those findings will find them in the Appendix.

Question 11 sought information about respondents' ethnic identifications. These data proved interesting. We have explained earlier why we did not analyze the responses of those marking "Native American" on the form. Although more than 75% of the responses were from those identifying themselves as Caucasian, it was possible to make some analysis of how Hispanics and African Americans differed from the majority.

One day a leader of a local breast cancer support group made the casual comment that although there were a number of African American women in her groups, she could not think of any who had implants. We called another support group organizer who told us the same thing. We then began to ask plastic surgeons if any of their implant patients were African American, and the answer was "no." Were these reports idiosyncratic or was there a systematic difference in values and perceptions?

Figure 9.2 compares responses of African American and Caucasian subjects on a number of items on our survey and shows both differences and similarities. Both ethnic groups were very familiar with the issue on Item 1. Both use print and broadcast media heavily, but Caucasians were more likely to report using newspapers and broadcast news and less likely to report using talk shows.

Because the number of African Americans is small, the difference needed for statistical significance at the .05 level was not achieved, but the two groups differed on 10 of the 21 attitude items by at least .4 of a point. The pattern of these items is interesting. All but one of the differences reflect less positive attitudes toward implants by the African American respondents. Only on Item 3m, "implants make it harder to detect breast cancer," were they more positive. On Items 4 and 5, African Americans reported themselves as much less likely to advise breast implants. On Items 6 and 7, they were less likely to know someone with implants or to have them

1.	Heard about implants—	
	African Americans:	12 yes 1 no
	Caucasians:	294 yes 3 no

2. Information Sources—
African Americans use less:
newspapers   62% vs. 79%
broadcastnews   77% vs. 96%
African Americans use more:
talk shows   62% vs. 55%

3. Attitude items with at least a .4 scaling point difference—
African Americans agree more:
  a. Most women will get sick   3.27 vs. 2.82
  b. Most implants leak   3.33 vs. 2.81
  d. Manufacturers covered up re: danger   4.42 vs.4.04
  n. Women with implants must accept
    whatever happens   3.08 vs. 2.58
  o. Women would be smart to have them out   3.58 vs. 2.99
African Americans disagree more:
  e. Implant danger has been exaggerated   2.25 vs. 2.70
  g. Women with implants
    feel better about themselves   3.67 vs. 4.09
  i. Implants truly needed postmastectomy   2.83 vs.3.35
  m. Implants make it hard to detect breast cancer   3.08 vs. 3.57

		African Americans	Caucasians
4.	I would advise implants following breast removal due to cancer	9 %	39%
5.	I would advise implants in order to look better	0%	12%
6.	Knows someone who has implants	58%	67%
7.	Has implants	0%	6%
8.	Mean age	37	40
9.	Mean income of you and spouse	$37,000	$55,000

FIG. 9.2. How African Americans differ from Caucasians
on the implant survey.

	Hispanic		African American		Caucasian	
	yes	no	yes	no	yes	no
1. Heard about implants	15	0	12	1	294	3
2. Sources of information						
Newspapers	80%		61%		79%	
Broadcast news	93%		77%		93%	
Talk shows	67%		62%		55%	
Friends	27%		46%		50%	
Doctor or nurse	20%		8%		11%	
3. Items with a .4 difference						
3a Most women get sick	3.53				2.82	
3b Most implants leak	3.47				2.81	
3d Makers covered up	4.60				4.04	
3e Danger exaggerated	2.20				2.76	
3g Women feel better	4.07				3.67	
3m Hard to detect cancer	3.73				3.08	
3r Implants are safe	1.87		2.50		2.35	
3t Most replaced	3.60		3.18			
3u If safe I'd consider	2.20		1.42			
4. I'd advise implants postmastectomy	13%		9%		39%	
5. I'd advise implants in order to look better	13%		0%		12%	
6. Know woman with implants	73%		58%		67%	
7. Has implants	7%		0%		6%	
8. Mean age	31		37		40	
9. Mean income you and your spouse	$37,000		$37,000		$55,000	
10. Respondents	15		13		297	

FIG. 9.3. Differences among Hispanics, African Americans, and Caucasians.

themselves. These results indicate that implants are a less important part of the lives of African Americans and that they regard them less favorably than do Caucasians.

The responses of Hispanics follow a still different pattern. They are like and unlike both African Americans and Caucasians. Figure 9.3 makes the comparisons. Hispanics have heard about the issue just as the others have. Like Caucasians, they used newspapers and broadcast news as sources, but Hispanics' use of talk shows is more frequent, similar to African Americans. They did not use conversations with friends as much as either of the other two groups, but they talked about the issue with doctors and nurses nearly twice as much as either Caucasians or African Americans.

Hispanics' responses to the attitude items follow an interesting pattern. Their responses are stronger concerning the risks of implants. They agree more strongly than Caucasians that "most women will get sick," "most implants will leak," and that "manufacturers covered up information." They disagree more strongly than Caucasians that "implant danger has been exaggerated" and that "implants are safe." They agree more strongly than African Americans that "implants make it harder to detect cancer," and that "most implants will have to be replaced." They disagree more that "implants are safe."

Given these perceptions that implant risks are higher, one would expect Hispanics to be more negative about implants. But they are not. More strongly than African Americans, they agree that women with implants "feel better about themselves," and that "if implants were safe they would consider having them." Their average score for considering having implants is 2.20 compared to 1.42 for African Americans, 1.89 for Caucasians, and 1.91 overall. Despite the greater intensity of their feelings about risks, they are more likely to consider having implants.

Perhaps this is because they also feel more intensely about the benefits. Hispanics are less likely to recommend implants after a mastectomy, but more likely to recommend them for cosmetic purposes. Indeed, they do not make the differentiation between the two purposes the way other subjects do. They are more likely to know someone with implants, but no more likely to have them. Their willingness to consider implants despite their belief in the risks may well reflect the power of benefits to influence risk taking. In our discussion of communication and risk in other chapters, we considered the idea that people are risk aversive only in regard to loss and danger, but they are willing to take risks in proportion to their belief in the possibility of gain. This hypothesis explains gambling, among other types of behavior. Hispanic women may be more willing to consider implants because they believe more strongly in the potential benefits.

CONCLUSIONS

Our survey of 400 Tampa Bay area women in the early summer of 1992 provides an interesting glimpse of how those similar to potential implant recipients responded to the intense publicity about the controversy over silicone gel breast implants. This was not an issue that escaped their attention. Nearly 99% had encountered information about the controversy.

The only source that had strong influence on attitudes was whether a respondent had talked to a doctor or nurse about the topic. If they had, they were more favorable about the risks and benefits of implants, as well as about the people involved. Those women who relied solely on media sources of information were the most negative about implants. We believe this is a direct reflection of the predominant use of the narrative paradigm in media coverage of danger, contrasted with the use of the rational paradigm in presenting material about safety (see chap. 6 on the media coverage).

The attitude items in our survey that elicited the strongest reactions, in either the agreement or disagreement direction, were those that described characters acting. They were, in a sense, mininarratives. We believe this observation adds support to the argument for the power of narrative discourse to persuade.

Those who themselves had implants were decidedly more favorable toward the safety and benefits of implants, and toward the characters in the controversy. Those who knew someone with implants were also more favorable about the risks and benefits. African American women were more negative about implants than the others, and were less willing to consider having them. Hispanic women by contrast, were more negative about the risks of implants than others, but more positive about their benefits as well. They were more likely than other women to consider having implants.

A perceived connection between health, breasts, and cancer emerged from our findings. Women see these as linked, despite the fact that media narratives did not focus primarily on cancer and implants. We attribute this finding to the deep concern about cancer among women that also became clear in our interviews with women with implants. Even though there was less public debate about cancer as a risk of implants than about other health risks, women believed more strongly that cancer was a problem for women with implants. More attention to this concern would have served the female public well, particularly because reassuring evidence is available.

The respondents in our survey were supportive of women who had chosen to have implants. They reserved their criticism for those they believe should protect their health—manufacturers, doctors, and the FDA.

Finally, our respondents showed measured judgment about the safety of implants. Although they refused to see them as safe, they also rejected most of the charges against implants. Women in the Tampa Bay area responded with considerable caution in drawing conclusions on an important medical issue about which disagreement exists among health authorities, and toward which little systematic scientific investigation had been directed at the time of the survey. Even with increasing support for safety claims, such caution seems prudent. Disputes still remain over frequency of ruptures and hardening, degree of risk for connective tissue diseases, and links to more subjective ailments.

APPENDIX 1

Attitudes of Demographic Groups

Age. Items 8 through 12 request demographic information. Responses to Item 10 did not prove to be useful. When tested to see if age made a difference in the use of information sources, we found one significant difference. Talk shows were selected as a source of information about implants more by women between 30 and 50 than those older and younger (chi-square (4) = 13.1, $p < .02$). Although the size of the differences did not reach the .05 level, there were direct linear differences according to age in the use of newspapers and broadcast news programs. The oldest women used both most and the youngest least. On three of the attitude items, age made a significant difference. On Item 3a, "most women with implants will get sick," mean agreement levels decreased linearly with age ($p < .01$). On Item 3b, "most implants leak," women above 50 agreed less than those below 50 ($p < .01$). On Item 3e, "implant danger had been exaggerated," agreement increases linearly with age ($p < .01$). There is some minimal evidence that the older women are, the less negative they are about implants.

Income. Only two attitude items showed an influence of income level. On Item 3r, "implants are safe," agreement is higher for those with incomes between $40,000 and $80,000 than for those higher and lower ($p < .05$). On Item 3t, "most implants will have to replaced," the greatest agreement was for those under $40,000 and above $80,000 ($p < .02$). These differences do not seem to offer a meaningful pattern.

Education. On only two items did education level make a significant difference. Those with more education were significantly more likely to list newspapers (chi-square (4) = 11.99, $p < .02$) and broadcast news (chi-square (4) = 16.45, $p < .01$) as information sources. Mean agreement decreases linearly as education increases on Item 3n, "women with implants must accept whatever happens to them" ($p < .01$).

Overall, although there are some differences according to these demographic variables, they did not account for strong overall differences in the results of our survey.

10

INTERPRETING THE STORIES: LESSONS FOR COMMUNICATING ABOUT HEALTH

We began this project because two plastic surgeons wondered about the ethics of removing implants, a medical procedure that involved risk, without having a perceived health benefit. As we talked with our surgeon colleagues and between ourselves, we generated a cluster of related questions: What are acceptable reasons for implant removal? Who is empowered to make that decision? What reasons do women have for wanting their implants removed? How did the motivation for removal eclipse the initial motivation to have implants? What if patients and physicians do not share ideas about scientific justification for implant removal? How have women been influenced in their decision making about implants and removal? Do women who want their implants removed differ in their analysis of risk from women who are satisfied with their implants? Who has a choice of what medical procedures a patient elects?

As we explored these questions in the previous nine chapters, we found our attention continually drawn to several important issues involved in how patients make decisions and the kinds of information on which those decisions are based: What happens when scientific debate occurs in public forums? How does information about therapeutic risk influence decision making? How does the doctor-patient relationship relate to the public debate and to patients' understanding of risk information? We have discussed these questions and offered possible answers throughout this book. Those answers generally point in the direction of complexity rather than simplicity. As much as we might like answers to be clear and simple, most are not. In examining the question of differing opinions on implants by differing medical specialties in chapter 5, for example, we could not conclude that one group held the truth and the other was in error. Rather, we suggested that multiple issues contribute to the different conclusions that specialists reach and the contradictory advice they give to patients: the nature of the specialists' practices, the presence of referral bias, and the way clinical knowledge is related to scientific inquiry. We invite the reader to review the conclusions already offered in each chapter to see this complexity emerge.

The concept of narrative, both as a method of investigation and as a feature of discourse, provided the perspective through which this complexity was revealed. The use of narrative analysis has allowed us to consider multiple influences and situational elements that affected women, physicians, the press, drug manufacturers, and the public concerning the safety and efficacy of breast implants. The competing stories provide us with a renewed "appreciation [for] the tangled swirl of emotions, relationships, power dynamics, diversions, resources, bureaucratic constraints and happenstance in ethical decision making" (Brown, 1993, p. 3). As we consider the way patients' stories, physicians' experiences, media accounts, public relations strategies, and public reactions emerged, we can see the complexity of medical decision making as a process where public discussion and personal relationships intertwine. One of the most intriguing issues is how scientific information plays out in public media.

PUBLIC USES OF SCIENTIFIC INFORMATION

The Media Context for Health Care Messages

Clearly, the media played an enormous role in women's, physicians', and the public's understanding, attitudes, and decisions concerning implants. Chapter 6 demonstrates the enormous coverage that television, newspapers, and magazines gave to the issue. Chapters 4 and 5 describe the blame that physicians and satisfied women attributed to media sensationalism of health risks. Chapter 3 explains how sick women used the media to fulfill their needs for explanation, control, and connection. Our opinion poll confirmed the news as the primary source of public information about the controversy.

Although physicians expressed frustration about the amount of media coverage given to what they believed was minimal risk affecting a very small number of unsatisfied patients, they should not have been surprised. The breast implant controversy included five issues that can be used to predict a high level of public controversy about the regulation of medical care, creating a popular media forum for scientific discourse: (a) the widespread public use of the implants, (b) the high political importance of the implant makers, (c) the economic importance of the implants, (d) a considerable public attachment to implants and what they represent, and (e) a low shared public understanding about the risks involved in the procedure (Bantz, 1981). Clearly, plastic surgery is a lucrative field for physicians and generates millions of dollars for the medical industry. Just as clearly, the controversy played out as a confrontation between the regulatory power of the FDA and one of the most powerful drug companies in the world. The fact that millions of women have implants heightened public and media attention. More detailed examination of the latter two issues reveals some of the most important relationships we discovered in our study.

The Issue Raised Public Controversy and Significant Media Attention Because it Focused On a Product With a High Social Value

Bantz (1981) argued that when the government attempts to restrict the use of a drug, food, or product that has high value for the public, the regulatory action is likely to cause considerable controversy and generate significant media coverage. In the case of breast implants, the device represented a tension in public values concerning appearance and substance.

Plastic surgery is caught in a fundamental value conflict in our society over the question of form and content. Breast implants and other cosmetic surgery represent a schism in some of our most fundamental social values. Our folk traditions tell us to watch out for the fast talker, the insincere lover, the glib suitor, and the false prophet, all of whom trade on appearing to be something they are not. We are taught to look inside people to find true substance and not to be deceived by superficial appearance.

But as a society we take appearance very seriously. We are good at slogans, packaging, and makeup. We pursue fashion vigorously and discard clothing, not when it is worn out, but when it goes out of style. We have our bodies wrapped, our nails manicured, and our hair styled. Young executives are counseled on how to dress for success. Both sexes spend millions on deodorants, scent, and hair spray. It is axiomatic in the social sciences that first impressions are lasting impressions. We take great care in how we appear. But even as we select our stationery carefully and make sure our shoes are shined, we worry that preoccupation with appearance reflects only vanity and the shallowest of values. We are distrustful of our own vanity at the same time that we are driven by it.

Surely, the role we ascribe to the female breast exhibits this conflict. No one of any sense would argue that a woman's contribution to society, her desirability as a friend, her ability as a professional, her value as a wife, her skill as a lover, or even her ability to nurse a child, is dependent on having large breasts.

Yet, we act as if breast size does matter. Some men joke about breast size using a variety of well-known euphemisms. Lingerie manufacturers successfully market garments designed to make breasts more prominent. The Wonder Bra is news. There are books and articles in women's magazines about how to have more beautiful breasts. Exercise aids and creams are sold as breast-enlarging agents. They sell, despite evidence that they do not and cannot work, because appearance matters and the hope of improving appearance is powerful.

In an episode of *Designing Women,* Mary Jo comments about the attention she is receiving from men when wearing a set of falsies, "These things are real power." We laugh because falsies cannot be the source of power; all the while knowing that they do make a difference. Dolly Parton's bust line provides a thousand punch lines for comedians, but millions admire her, and she laughs all the way to the bank. Big breasts should not be important: character should; intelligence should; spirit should; kindness should; skill should; unselfishness should; ability should. But "should" is not "does." Substantive concerns do not always, maybe even usually, carry the day. Appearance matters, even if a part of us would like to subordinate it to substance.

The women we interviewed knew their value was not in their breasts, but their motives for implant surgery were compelling, nonetheless. Women who sought reconstructive surgery following mastectomies did not feel whole or normal until they regained the female appearance that disease took from them. Women who had augmentation surgery felt tangible pain as a result of being small chested in a society where breast size matters. The proposed regulations and investigations over the safety of implants were the focus of significant public controversy and media coverage, in part, because breast implants epitomize our cultural value on appearance and the conflict we feel about the ways we fulfill that value.

The Issue Was Controversial Because of Low Shared Public Understanding of Risks

The implant issue also drew significant media coverage because of widespread confusion about side effects. According to Bantz (1981), when "low shared [public] understanding and high controversy intersect [they] . . . provide the conditions for an argumentative free-for-all" (p. 75). Four elements contributed to public confusion over risks: (a) a lack of balance between risks and benefits, (b) the combination of known and unknown risks, (c) the failure to distinguish between types of implants and attendant side effects, and (d) previous underrepresentation of implant risks. All of these elements were compounded by inherent problems in arguing science in a public forum.

Media Reports Failed to Provide Information About Benefits and Risks Proportionate to Their Likelihood of Occurrence.   Even though all the physicians we spoke to agreed that serious health risks for implants were low, the media gave much more attention to a wide variety of serious health risks than to the benefits of the medical device. Physicians argued that news reports distorted risks, confused the public about scientific evidence of safety, and ignored health benefits.

Clearly, there was no shared public understanding about the amount of risk that the implants posed to women who had them. Yet, the implant controversy was not a unique phenomenon in media discussions about health risks and scientific information. News reports do not usually include information about risks and benefits proportionate to their likelihood of occurrence. The absence of such a perspective is characteristic of media reporting on health issues. Singer and Endreny's (1993) review of media reports of risk indicates that media news focuses primarily on risks; very little on benefits. Conversely, Molitor (1983) reported that when the *New England Journal of Medicine* published a study concerning the benefits of aspirin to prevent heart attack, news media minimized the risks associated with the treatment. Whether the news underrepresents risks or benefits in individual cases, it appears that the media are not good at placing risks in perspective for the public.

For the press, a story has news value if it presents the unusual or the dramatic. A careful attempt to explain the complex nature of risk does not make good news, but a patient's suffering is news even if it is not likely to happen to others. People cannot rely on health news to tell them how to assess health risks and plan sensible health behavior.

The breast implant controversy was no exception. Neither television, nor magazines, nor newspapers provided readers with relative or absolute standards by which to measure risks of the procedures. Often the only probability measurements were the reporters' qualifiers: "The FDA will announce this week that the most popular type of implant . . . presents women with an *unacceptably high risk* of cancer" (Friedman, 1991a; emphasis added) or "leakage of silicone *may* cause autoimmune disease or even cancer" (Friedman, 1991b; emphasis added). A very few times, the news provided the public with an assessment of relative risks by comparing implant removal to keeping them, "for now risk of cancer or birth defects [from implants] appears *so small* that women should not have their implants removed" (Sorenson, 1991; emphasis added). However, news media provided no anchors on which women could base comparisons of risk.

Media Reports Mixed Known and Unknown Risks.   Contributing to public confusion was the combination of side effects that media associated with breast implants. The controversy grew in ambiguity because of the mixing of known and uncertain risks that were not distinguished consistently in public discourse. Sick women and the media reported several symptoms physicians clearly acknowledged as caused by the implants: ruptures, leaks and bleeding, hardening, implant migration, and granulomas. Other risks were clearly related to problems inherent in any surgery: postsurgical infections and scarring. These, too, were acknowledged by physicians. The only controversy over these symptoms appeared to be about the percentage of women likely to experience them.

Although there was disagreement among physicians about the existence and likelihood of autoimmune disease and almost unanimous agreement that cancer was not a risk, these diseases were often grouped with known risks of leakage, ruptures, and hardening. NBC related, "The FDA spelled out the dangers this past week: hardening . . . silicone leakage through the body, and an increased risk of cancer" (Gould & Zucker, 1991). Six months later the network report included multiple problems: "They can break or leak. Silicone may spread through the body and may cause serious stiffening of joints or stiffening of skin. In animal tests, silicone can cause cancer. The new breast may harden or lose its shape" (Gould & Zucker, 1992b). In January, NBC reported:

> Senior FDA officials are calling the implant decision their toughest in years. Arguing the devices can rupture, leaking silicone into the body causing cancer or autoimmune joint diseases, critics point to 5,000 complaints of side effects over the last 8 years. (Gould & Zucker, 1992a)

News reports consistently linked known risks (ruptures, leakage, hardening) with unknown or disputed risks (autoimmune diseases and cancer). It is reasonable to assume that, when the media fail to distinguish one risk from another and engage in clumping, as we saw earlier, that the public is encouraged to see the risks as similar and similarly established. At the very least, the media reporting discouraged individuals from sorting known from unknown side effects.

One of the most troubling consequences of mixing side effects is the media representation of cancer risk. As noted in chapter 5, all the physicians we spoke to indicated that they found no relationship between having implants and an increased risk of cancer. Indeed, recent studies confirm that (Berkel et al., 1992). Surprisingly, of the 70 side effects listed in media accounts, the risk of cancer was among the top five most frequently mentioned. Although cancer was not a part of the individual women's horror stories, it was often listed among specific harms from the narratives. The association of cancer with dramatically told accounts, clumped a dreaded disease with other lesser risks that were acknowledged to occur, at least part of the time. The fact that the Alberta study (Berkel et al., 1992) received relatively little coverage despite its power to reassure those worried about implants causing cancer, illustrates the preoccupation by the press with danger rather than safety.

Media Reports Did Not Distinguish Between Risks of Specific Types of Implants.   The reporting of cancer risk was further problematized by early reports of the Même and Replicon implants, which had polyurethane covers. FDA reports that poly covers broke down into TDA, an animal carcinogen, led to a withdrawal of the implants from the market. Early reports on the implant controversy focused heavily on the cancer connection to TDA. For example, television news reported the link between polyurethane and TDA in almost every news segment in our collection from December 1990 through November 1991 (10 out of 12 news segments). No research was ever done to show that the coating would break down yielding that chemical in humans and/or that it would affect people as it did laboratory animals. Instead, the Même implant was withdrawn from the market. Although the poly-coated implants were removed from the market in April 1991, news reports of a cancer risk continued throughout the controversy, very often without direct reference to the poly-coated implants, but ascribed to silicone gel implants in general. Toward the end of 1992, news coverage focused on concerns of implants blocking mammogram screening.

Even though the poly-coated implants were removed from the market in 1991, reports throughout the news coverage referred to cancer as one of the "possible side effects" (Gross, 1991, p. A1), advised that there was "considerable reason to suspect" cancer is linked to implants (Rovner, 1991, p. 6), and warned that the "possible long term effects" of implants include cancer ("Overreaction to Implant Controversy," 1992, p. 3A).

The news accounts raised concern about a cancer risk by associating unknown risks with known ones, and by mixing news of specific cancer risks (poly–coated implants and concerns over mammograms) with warnings applied to implants in general. The failure to specify and distinguish risks increased the likelihood that audiences would attribute cancer risks to all silicone implants, without distinguishing between types. In addition, the primacy and recency phenomenon also contribute to the memory of the cancer risk. We remember those concepts that are presented first and last in speeches, events, and written documents. In this case, the implant controversy began with news about TDA and ended with concerns over implants blocking views in mammograms. It is likely that those issues are the best remembered by the public.

Chapter 9 indicated that women we surveyed linked silicone breast implants to cancer. Indeed, the risk to which subjects reacted most strongly was the risk of cancer. The mixing of cancer risks with known risks, the failure to distinguish between types of implants, and the primacy-recency phenomenon are very likely to be responsible for part of the association.

The Media Encouraged a Perception That Plastic Surgeons and Manufacturers Had Historically Underrepresented Risks. One other element of the media stories could have increased public belief in cancer risk, as well as autoimmune disease—the perception that physicians and manufacturers had underestimated the known implant risks in the past. Plastic surgeons often reported known risks as less likely to occur than the media described. Doctors we talked to cited studies indicating that ruptures or infection were likely in only 6 to 12% of cases. However, almost every media narrative about sick women included an account of one or more ruptures. One third of the women we talked to had suffered ruptures or leaks. Media included reports in which one third of the women considered had suffered ruptures or leakage and stated that "all the devices 'bleed' . . . some components of the silicone leak through the enclosing sac" (Seligmann & Church, 1992, p. 75).

Media stories encouraged a perception that plastic surgeons and manufacturers had, at best, underestimated known risks, and at worst, had lied. When reporting Dow's ½ % rupture figure, newspapers cited scientists who said the drug company's estimates were 10 times lower than FDA figures. The reports sometimes implied that the risks had been hidden: "Documents obtained earlier by the FDA from Dow Corning Corporation, the leading implant maker, show that in the past 15 years it had received reports from several individual doctors that up to 32 percent of their implant patients suffered ruptures" (Hilts, 1992c, p. 12A). Dow's ½ % rupture figures were compared with the FDA statement that "implants should not be relied upon for a lifetime" and that "women should be prepared [to have them] replaced" ("Panel Advises," 1992, p. 2A).

The reports encouraged the perception that Dow and plastic surgeons either did not know or had hidden the higher risk of implant ruptures. Public awareness of underrepresented known risks has implications for perceptions of disputed risks. News reports that manufacturers and plastic surgeons underestimated known risks were likely to influence public perceptions of other risks that the companies and doctors were denying. If they lied or did not know about the higher percentage of ruptures or leaks in the past, the company and plastic surgeons could be lying or unaware of cancer risks now.

Risk assessment of cancer and autoimmune disease might also have been affected by media stories that portrayed the history of implants as a series of initial safety assurances, subsequent discovery of harm, and eventual withdrawal of products and techniques as unsafe (told in chapter 7). If the scientific and medical community had often been wrong previously when it reassured women about enclosed capsulatomies, the Natural Y implants, and the polyurethane-coated implants, the public was likely to look on contemporary reassurances with skepticism. The reports about cancer and autoimmune risks in the early 1990s played out in a larger historical context of medical reversals about implant safety.

The question of breast cancer risks is particularly troubling because of our interviewees' intense fear of breast cancer. Women like Rachel and Elizabeth underwent preventive mastectomies to avoid cancer deaths and were especially sensitive to suggestions of a breast cancer link. Indeed, both of them chose saline implants before the ban on silicone.

Inherent Problems in Arguing Science in a Public Forum

The amount of public controversy and media coverage in the breast implant controversy illustrates that arguing science in the public arena is extremely difficult, particularly when audience members are laypersons. Bantz's study of public arguments over banning saccharin concluded that "the majority of the public had no way of judging the scientific quality of the [study linking saccharin to cancer], nor did the public accept the inevitability of regulation when they did not understand the rationale [against saccharin]" (1981, p. 79). Bantz's conclusion about saccharin holds true for the implant controversy as well. Most laypersons, including patients, have difficulty understanding health probabilities and translating them into the effect on their individual lives (Morris, 1990, p. 19).

The working procedures of scientific inquiry are also alien to the general public. Most people are not good at maintaining a posture of doubt, phrasing questions so they are subject to falsification, entertaining contrary hypotheses, understanding that the null hypotheses can only be rejected and not affirmed, considering sample size, using the law of large numbers, interpreting statistical significance, understanding the significance of regression toward the mean, reading data tables and graphs, or admitting previous error. The importance of waiting for a pattern of findings from both replication and a variety of approaches before drawing firm conclusions is difficult for a public who want immediate and definite answers. What is a compelling story to reporter and reader, is to the scientist an individual account with significant potential to mislead until the case is supported by large controlled studies. The media reports in our sample did little to clarify scientific process.

We think that people are most influenced by those individual cases in the form of narratives. The concept of recall bias reinforces public reliance on risk narratives:

To make a decision, patients must recall pertinent information bearing on the decision and then evaluate those factors. However . . . not all the information bearing upon [a] decision is "available" in memory. Only the most vivid and salient information is likely to be recalled. Pallid statistical data based upon a large number of experiences may be disregarded in lieu of a more vivid personal experience with one case. In addition, negative information may be more distinct than positive information and more easily recalled. A patient who knows of one person having had a negative experience with a therapy may fail to remember reading a favorable report. (Morris, 1990, pp. 92-93)

Not only are dramatic accounts more likely to be recalled when they are personal experiences, but also when they are on the news (Singer & Endreny, 1993). Bantz (1981) argued that the power of dramatic themes extends beyond the enhancement of memory. His saccharin study demonstrated the triumph of dramatic narrative themes over scientific expertise and accuracy (1981). As we finish this last chapter, the Supreme Court has refused to hear arguments by Dow Corning that testimony in Mariann Hopkins' 1991 trial was not based on scientific principles ("Breast Implant Award," 1995) and two rheumatologists have resigned from panels to study silicone risks because they previously consulted for drug companies ("Doctors Resign," 1994). The perceived ethics of the players continues to be more important in public decision making than the discussion of scientific process. Chapter 9 confirms the focus on narrative elements; the public responded more strongly to issues about characters than about the scientific elements in the controversy.

The public's response to narrative, rather than rational argument, complicates the decision-making process for physicians, patients, and regulators. If science is our best source of information about health and the efficacy of health behavior, but we fail to understand or respond to the rhetoric of scientific processes, how can we, collectively as a society and individually, make intelligent health decisions? Rational discourse does not persuade, particularly scientific discourse, with its special demands. Science is an achievement in the domains where we can make it work precisely because it does not fit ordinary ways of thinking and acting.

If society still trusted experts, we could accept scientific conclusion on the basis of authority. However, we no longer trust experts. In the case of the breast implant controversy, media accounts undermined the credibility of plastic surgeons and drug manufacturers; the two groups in the best position to evaluate the safety and efficacy of implants. The press routinely juxtaposes what are presented as equally competent experts either to balance a report or to get a controversial story (depending on one's perspective on press ethics). News media often show the layperson challenging the expert, fulfilling a familiar David and Goliath plotline, with the audience cheering David. When the expert tries to respond using scientific discourse, he or she often fails, because the public does not understand data the way the scientist does. And of course, scientists can be self-serving just like everyone else.

This may be a benign problem as long as we are talking about quantum mechanics or even the design of jet aircraft where individuals are not called on to make decisions. But in health care we want to communicate about risks and benefits, so people can make good decisions. What is the expert on health communication to advise? Do not give data, just stories? Teach the public about science? Maybe both?

Asking health professionals to communicate through narratives will be challenging because we know doctors value abstract exposition over anecdotes; our interviews tell us that. But narratives are the substance of media, and this is the stuff that most conveys benefits and risks in the public arena. Doctors need to be able to develop dramatic stories of safety and efficacy if they are hoping to contribute to public discussions of risk.

The Interplay of Narratives in Public Discussion and Private Decisions

Even when we consider the public's propensity to understand the world and health information through a narrative perspective, we still have to grapple with why some stories chained out in the media and others did not. Why did the horror stories play out so heavily in the media, serve as such a potent force in the sick women's medical decisions, and become reflected in our public opinion poll? Eraker, Kirscht, and Becker (1984) explained that health decisions are made based on multiple influences, including our general health beliefs, our relationship with medical personnel, our past history with health professionals, and our support networks. We believe that the horror stories, with their attendant vilification of plastic surgeons, were persuasive and chained through the press—rather than stories of supportive physicians, happy women, and implant benefits described in chapters 4 and 5—because the horror stories included familiar narrative themes. The characterizations of women as victims, plastic surgeons as villains, and drug companies as profit-hungry big businesses, were complementary to other contemporary cultural stories and beliefs about health and the medical community.

The horror story is congruent with increased perception and awareness of danger and a growing disillusionment with physicians; "Throughout the 1970s, numerous health disasters, a multitude of health warnings, and a marked politicization of public health issues transformed our sense of safety" (Crawford, 1984, p. 74). The perception of danger has only increased since Crawford's commentary. Recent publicity about a surgeon who amputated a diabetic patient's wrong foot or the nurse who turned off the respirator of the wrong patient is part of the larger web of narratives about errors and misjudgments in health care. They are told in news stories and repeated in our interpersonal conversations about the risks of modern medical care. The counternarrative about the doctor cutting off the diseased foot is not news precisely because it almost always happens, but that absence from the press reports fails to give reassurance or a perspective on risk.

The news media routinely report that drug companies fail to disclose risks of their products to the FDA. During the height of the implant controversy, the media described violations by Lily, Upjohn, and Phizer. The implant story played out in a context that the FDA was under fire for failing to protect the public, the controversy "can only serve to cast more doubt on the FDA's ability to do its job [protect the public]" (Friedman, 1992).

The horror story was also believable because it was congruent with other much publicized and highly visible syndromes. Sick women with multiple, unexplained symptoms, which they attributed to implants, told stories about being ignored by the medical community. The symptoms of Gulf War syndrome sounded much like the implant stories—muscle pain, memory loss, birth defects, respiratory ailments, heart problems, and cancer. The reaction of the medical community to Gulf War syndrome resonated with the sick women's stories of doctors' reactions to silicone connective tissue disorder. Physicians stated that most of those complaining of Gulf War syndrome had other illnesses that explained their symptoms.

As in silicone disease, the medical community claimed that no concrete evidence existed leading to the conclusion that a single disease caused the multiple symptoms. Similar to the implant controversy, a powerful agency, the federal government, denied culpability for the veterans' problems. Affected veterans claimed their ailments were linked to chemical warfare or measures the government required of veterans to protect U.S. troops. As in the implant story, only a small but vocal group has been affected ("Research on Gulf War," 1995; Cowley, Hager, & Liu, 1994).

Reinforcing stories of medical misdiagnosis in the implant controversy is increasing news coverage of Marfan's syndrome, "a disorder of the connective tissue" the syndrome is "often misdiagnosed or undetected" (Gosier, 1995, p. 1B). Like silicone tissue disorder stories, doctors frequently attribute Marfan's symptoms to other causes and are described as ignorant about the disease. Columnist Elijah Gosier described his brother's illness: "My brother spent much of the last few years of his life teaching the doctors who were treating him about the illnesses." Similar to the silicone problem, "there is no specific laboratory test for it." For people who have it "finding the right doctor is a major concern" (Gosier, 1995, p. 1B). Individuals with Marfan's syndrome have developed local support groups and national foundations, similar to Command Trust and the Silicone Sisters that help patients deal with the problem and find rare doctors who understand and will help.

Recent news coverage has also been given to Multiple Chemical Sensitivity, a controversial ailment. Some doctors say it's psychological. Among those who consider it a physical disorder, there is disagreement over what causes it, how to define it, and how to treat it ("For Her," 1994, p. 4A). The symptoms vary but may include: "rashes, sinus problems, headaches, fatigue, gastrointestinal upsets, exaggerated sense of smell, wheezing, coughing, sore throat, and impaired memory or concentration" ("For Her," 1994, p. 4A). Like silicone disease, individuals who believe they suffer from this mysterious syndrome have found help in advocacy groups: the Human Ecology Action League, the National Center for Environmental Health Strategies, and the International Institute of Research for Chemical Hypersensitivity.

Clearly, the public and the women involved in the implant controversy are hearing and reading reports in which other syndromes not recognized within the larger medical community are named and described (Cowley et al., 1994). While physicians discount diseases that defy differential diagnosis, women are hearing and reading about syndromes reified in the press. When doctors tell women they are imagining their ailments, the patients can affirm their illnesses through comparisons with other syndromes, which are characterized by a variety of seemingly unrelated symptoms, and about which patients have to teach their physicians.

The sick women's horror stories that reached the media did not play out in isolation. Awareness of other illness stories provided the public with narratives that reinforced the elements of the media horror stories. These are stories in which doctors do not appear omniscient. The narratives confirm the patients', not the physicians' experiences. As a result, increasing numbers of patients are likely to challenge physicians with information gained by the media and are less willing to accept the physicians' interpretations if it conflicts with individual experience, media accounts, or both.

The horror stories combined not only with other media illness stories, but also with many patients' personal experiences. Sick women's accounts and media stories of hurried and profit-hungry doctors are congruent with growing perceptions about medical practitioners. The doctor who spent too little time with patients to give good advice rings true with many patients' experiences with physicians. A recent survey of 70,000 Americans identified lack of communication as characteristic of their relationships with their doctors ("How Is Your Doctor," 1995). Specifically, respondents reported that many physicians were not open to patients' questions, did not ask for patients' opinions, and did not give much information. The survey results reinforced findings over the past two decades of patients' growing concerns over doctors' perceived lack of concern and misdiagnosis (Korsch et al., 1968; Korsch & Negrete, 1972; Mechanic, 1968; Todd, 1989).

The stories also resonate with increased perception of the medical treatment of women in general. The fact that patients who receive breast implants are female is not insignificant in understanding public acceptance and media chaining of the sick women's stories. Women have recently begun to question medical practice in other ways. They have argued for the need for more women in what has been a masculine profession in both numbers and mind set. The frequency of hysterectomies, radical mastectomies, Caesarean deliveries, and psychiatric treatment for women has been challenged by the women's movement (Boston Women's Health Book Collective, 1984). The validity of criticism by women of the paucity of female subjects in medical research has been acknowledged by the CDC's recent initiative for research on women's health. At an individual level, women often report that doctors do not listen to them or take their complaints seriously. Women are more likely to receive mood–altering medications than men, often for symptoms for which men receive no prescriptions at all (Ogur, 1984).

For women whose own doctors have seemed to be poor listeners or in a hurry, these accounts will be believable. A number of women's current concerns about medicine are reflected in news accounts of the implant controversy because the stories seem to be one more case where women are victims of medicine men, with the accent on men.

THE PLACE OF RELATIONSHIPS IN MEDICAL DECISIONS

Although it is clear that media played a major role in presenting harms, heightening awareness of risk, and promoting a particular set of stories, our research suggests that the influence of the media is affected by relationships that women have with friends, family, and their physicians. Satisfied women consistently dismissed media reporting as sensationalism. Even those who had health problems that sick women attributed to their implants discounted the media reports if they had support systems that provided alternate explanations. From the importance that women placed on support networks, family, and friends as reference points for understanding their health, we can see that health decisions are made within the context of social communities, which are used as mirrors for women's experiences with their health. The public opinion poll confirmed the power of relationships over the media. Individuals who knew someone who had implants or had talked with medical personnel about them were less affected by media accounts than were those individuals who relied exclusively on the news reports. Personal contacts appear to be more powerful in health decisions and perceptions of health risks than are media accounts.

Even more primary to the women's decisions is the relationship they have with their physicians. In the breast implant controversy, doctors' and women's relationships broke down badly. Sick women blamed their physicians for misinformation and incompetence. Physicians blamed patients who were difficult, time consuming, and had psychological problems. The cycle of blame resulted in patients' perceptions of abandonment and a withdrawal from the medical care system. Physicians were unlikely to assume blame, but withdrew from angry patients. As a result, women felt abandoned by their doctors. Such blaming and withdrawal appears to exacerbate poor recovery; "One of the most consistent findings in the literature on adapting to threatening circumstances . . . [is that] believing that someone else is to blame is related to physical impairment and emotional distress" (Tennen & Affleck, 1990, p. 209).

Unfortunately, the tendency to find blame in situations where health is threatened seems to be a contemporary commonplace; "In a society like ours, the need to fix responsibility, to locate a cause and preferably an agent, is pervasive . . . . In such a culture the ultimate horror is a disaster without an explanation, an essentially random event" (Singer & Endreny, 1993, p. 104). For the sick women, finding a cause for the major disruption in their lives might be empowering; it helps them to cope. Such attributions might also rob them of the support of physicians who could help.

When patients blame their physicians or withdraw from medical care in anger, the repercussions for the doctor can also be significant and extend beyond professional frustration. They can be economically devastating. Studies identifying causes for legal suits against physicians include patients who are angry because their physicians failed to communicate risks, were perceived to have ignored the patient, or communicated a superior or hurried attitude toward the patient (Morris, 1990). Women who believe their implants made them sick blame their physicians for the very same reasons that patients are most likely to sue their doctors. Indeed, thousands of women have enrolled in class action suits against implant manufacturers and many others are suing individual physicians.

What can physicians learn from the implant controversy about the doctor–patient relationship? Several issues seem relevant. Research on patient satisfaction suggests that doctors who are patient-centered are less likely to be blamed by their patient for negative outcomes: "This approach . . . encourages doctors to include patients as partners in health care. It encourages patients to ask questions, to seek a second opinion, and to share responsibility for medical decisions" ("How Is Your Doctor," 1995, p. 82).

Patient–centered physicians share authority for decision making with their patients. Research on the doctor–patient relationship suggests that equalizing the power differential between doctors and patients decreases the likelihood that doctors will be blamed for negative outcomes:

> When an authority is involved in a threatening event, whether or not present at the time of the event, the probability of other-blame increases. For example, mothers of premature infants, who were under the care of their obstetrician at the time of the premature delivery, showed a high incidence of other-blame directed primarily toward the doctor . . . . Our prediction regarding the authority, knowledge, and ability of the other suggests that medical specialists may be at greater risk of being blamed than general practitioners for an untoward outcome. It also suggests that the more that experts exert their authority to engender compliance, the greater their risk of being blamed for a negative outcome . . . . If medical authorities can share the responsibility and the risks of care, they may be able to reduce the incidence of other-blame and its attendant suffering. (Tennen & Affleck, 1990, p. 220)

The women's narratives in chapters 3 and 4 are congruent with Tennen and Affleck's advice. Several of the satisfied women we talked to took control of their health care decisions early in their consideration of breast implants. Many carried out research independent of their physician's advice. Despite some medical complications following their implant surgery, the women who assumed initial responsibility for their health care decisions were less likely to be angry with their physicians than women described in chapter 3 who became stewards of their own health late in their stories. Even those women who were ill and blamed their implants for their ailments responded positively to physicians who worked to establish partnerships with them. Barbara praised her physicians for giving her choices and information, and for leaving decision making up to her. Jill continued to see her walk-in clinic doctor precisely because the physician was willing to learn about the disease process with her, even though the physician did not know what Jill had. The partnership that developed between Jill and her doctor was one of the striking results of sharing authority.

Stories from chapter 5 also support the efficacy of doctor–patient partnerships. Two plastic surgeons we talked to were proactive in sharing choices with their patients when the news of implant risks emerged. They called their patients and shared their opinion about minimal implant risks, but still offered to remove the implants free of charge. Each had only one request for removal.

Another reason that authority figures and perceived experts are frequently blamed for negative outcomes is because people expect them to anticipate threatening events or possible risks (Tennen & Afflect 1990). Such a conclusion suggests that physicians should share information about risks and side effects with patients more than they currently do. A long chronology of studies, including patient self-report, physician interviews, and observation studies, indicate that many physicians do not regularly share information about side effects and possible risks with their patients. Studies from the mid-1970s found "a startling lack of therapeutic advice provided to patients by the doctor or the medical staff" (Morris, 1990, p. 41). More recent studies found that about one third of the patients received precautionary information about treatments and that only about one fourth of the patients received information about possible side effects (Morris, 1990).

Many sick women in chapters 2 and 3 told us that physicians had not mentioned any side effects to silicone implants. Some of the satisfied women did not recall any discussion of risks. All the women we talked to indicated that physicians underestimated the likelihood of ruptures. Although our interviewees recalled events, they are consistent with patient recall studies from other treatments that estimate physicians vary widely on the amount of risk disclosure they do with patients.

Although patient recall studies include limitations based on fallibility of the human memory, Morris (1990) explained that patients also fabricate additional information "that is logically consistent with what they believe should have been delivered but was not actually provided" (p. 43). As a result, patients might have forgotten that physicians told them about risks and side effects. But they might also have reported that doctors gave them information that the patients actually did not receive.

Even in cases where physicians do attempt to provide a perspective on risk, they are unlikely to provide an anchor on which patients can base understanding of relative risks and to make decisions. Physicians usually provide risk information in the form of adjectives. The probability of side effects occurring may be described as rare, improbable, unlikely, or doubtful. "Even among physicians there is a wide variance in the interpretation of these terms" (Morris, 1990, p. 92).

If patients are not provided with an anchor or an absolute numerical basis for assessing risks, it is more difficult for them to create a personal meaning for their chances of the risk. In the case of breast implants, the public did not receive that information from the media, and they were unlikely to have received much, if anything, specific about risks from their physicians. When the women were led to expect good outcomes, they felt betrayed when implants ruptured, migrated, hardened, and/or became infected. For those in perfect health before the implant surgery, the unexpected and unexplained devastation to health experienced by the sick women created bewilderment, anger, and ultimately a villain. Alternately, those women who had remembered advanced warning about ruptures and hardening were more philosophical about them when they occurred. Women who had explanatory frameworks in which to place arthritis and feelings of chest pressure did not blame them on their implants or their plastic surgeons.

The advice to share more side effects runs counter to many physicians' noble motives for not disclosing risks. Doctors are concerned that giving information about unlikely side effects frightens patients unnecessarily (Morris, 1990). Some studies show that when patients are warned about side effects, they are likely to attribute to medical treatment symptoms that they would otherwise not link to a health regimen. Especially susceptible patients have been shown to experience side effects described by a physician even when the patient was taking a placebo (Morris, 1990). As a result, most physicians share information only about the risks and side effects most likely to occur (Morris, 1990).

Such rationales assume that patients want to know about risks in order to make decisions about how likely they are to incur a side effect. Yet, Morris concluded that most patients do not make medical decisions based on the probability of risks occurring. Instead, many patients want to know about risks, even those very unlikely to occur. With this information, patients determine what the outcome of the risk would be, and whether they could live with it. As a result, the patients use risk information, not only to determine likelihood of occurrence, but as a coping mechanism. They ask, "What is the worst outcome, and could I live with it if it occurred?"

With possible risks in mind, the patient can better understand symptoms if they occur and knows what to expect and how to anticipate problems. Just being able to interpret events makes people feel better about themselves and increases mastery (Morris, 1990). Anger often stems from violated expectations. Letting people know what to expect, even in remote possibilities, reduces the likelihood of anger and increases patients' feelings of control.

Beyond giving the patient information, we might advise that the physician become more patient-centered in conducting interviews with their patients. Instead of moving through a list of predetermined questions based on the physician's understanding of illness, the doctor can spend some time asking for the patient's story. What does the patient think is wrong? What has the patient has been doing to help himself or herself? Does the patient know anyone else with similar symptoms? What was that person's treatment and outcome? What does the patient know about the prospective risks, side effects, treatments? By spending time understanding the meaning the patient gives to his or her illness and the reference points the patient has available, the physician can build on, modify, correct, and relate the patient's meaning to the understanding the physician would like the patient to accept (Smith, 1993).

The more information, interaction, and perspectives shared between the doctor and patient, the more partnership is built. Individuals caught in threatening events are less likely to blame their partners for a negative outcome. Instead, they search for other causes (Tennen & Affleck, 1990). We saw that clearly in the satisfied women's stories. They had long-term relationships with physicians. Most chose plastic surgeons who spent significant amounts of time talking to them. Some were doctors' wives, and others were medical personnel. As a result, many had close relationships and shared perspectives with physicians. These "connexional experiences" can increase patients' sense of control, and hence, their feelings of satisfaction (Morris, 1990, p. 127). These women did not blame their physicians as the cause of their problems nearly as much as did the women who did not have sustained partnerships with their physicians.

The decision to share more authority with patients, discuss more risks, give patients more choices, accept more of the patients' interpretations, and share more decisions is "bucking centuries-old habits and traditions. The role of the doctor as an authority and sole keeper of medical information dates back to Hippocrates" ("How Is Your Doctor," 1995, p. 81). Yet, the implant controversy demonstrates that physicians may have little choice. Media accounts of the controversy displayed cracks in the monolithic picture of medical consensus, with specialists calling other doctors incompetent. When news reports show physicians disagreeing on a variety of syndromes and cures, the public increasingly understands that a variety of opinions exist about their care and increasingly seeks second opinions. Voluntary health organizations and self-help groups are clearly influential in patients' decisions. They also serve as a form of empowerment for many of the sick women, compensating for the loss of support the women felt when they withdrew from physicians' care or when their doctors abandoned them.

In addition, self-help health groups and voluntary health organizations are fulfilling many roles once reserved for physicians. With many patients expressing a desire to be more involved in their health care decisions, doctors will be increasingly under pressure to serve as resources, rather than as the final authority on patients' health (Hitti, 1994).

CONCLUSION

Our primary perspective in this book has been a narrative interpretation of various accounts of the implant controversy. We tried to understand diverse experiences and decisions through a narrative framework. We have found the perspective useful in seeing how medical decisions are placed in context, the different health beliefs of women with implants, and the competing stories of women and their physicians. In addition, we have considered how and what stories played out across a wider media context. The silicone breast implant controversy became, for women and the public, less of a scientific argument than a study of competing narratives from magazines, television, newspapers, support groups, plastic surgeons, rheumatologists, friends, and family. All these influences contribute to the general and specific health beliefs that influence medical decision making.

This study has confirmed theories that no single element leads patients or physicians to a particular health care decision. Through the doctors', patients', and media stories, we recognize multiple influences. General health beliefs about how illnesses are diagnosed, the hereditary nature of illnesses, the psychological derivation of disease, and the inherent risks of medical procedures played a major role in all our stories. Patients' willingness to seek medical help, to accept medical direction, and to accept varying degrees of responsibility for their health care decisions were also critical elements of the narratives. The relationships between patients and their doctors were compelling parts of the implant narratives, as were connections to family and support networks. The degrees to which the players relied on different sources of information and influence, moved decision makers to different conclusions in their accounts.

These elements of patient decision making—general and specific health beliefs, patient preferences, satisfaction with the doctor–patient relationship, and the patient's support system—have been a part of various models of patient decision making for 3 decades (Eraker, Kirscht, & Becker, 1984). The narrative approach to understanding health decisions and controversies enables us to merge them into a greater understanding of how the elements intersect.

Unlike the scientific perspective that focuses on knowing the world and explaining it, narrative approaches emphasize "how we talk about the world and [try] to deal with it" (Bochner, 1994, p. 29). Narrative perspectives are particularly useful in forums like the implant controversy where ambiguity and chance play a role (Bochner, 1994). Narrative analysis focuses on the meaning that patients give to their experience and works from that understanding to make decisions and take action. "Narrative knowing recalls and recasts experience into meaningful signposts and supports for ongoing action" (Conguergood, 1993, p. 337). For women with silicone gel breast implants, the meaning they make of their experience with doctors, their implants, and their support systems is central to the decisions they make about their appearance, their health, and implant removal. Even though the FDA has severely restricted silicone implants, millions of women are carrying the devices in their bodies. The implant controversy may have been settled publicly by the 1992 FDA ruling, but women who have the implants will be making health care decisions related to the implants for the rest of their lives. Their stories are still evolving.

REFERENCES

CHAPTER 1

Angell, M. (1992). Breast implants—Protection or paternalism? *New England Journal of Medicine*, *326*, 1695–1696.

Brooks, P. M. (1995). Silicone breast implantation: Doubts about the fears. *Medical Journal of Australia*, *162*, 432–434.

Bruning, N. (1992). *Breast implants: Everything you need to know*. Alameda, CA: Hunter House.

Burton, T. M. (1996, February 28). Breast-implant study is fresh fuel for debate. *Wall Street Journal*, p. B1, B4.

Council on Scientific Affairs. (1993). Silicone breast implants. *Journal of the American Medical Association, 270*, 2602–2606.

Fisher, J. C. (1992). The silicone controversy—When will science prevail? *New England Journal of Medicine, 326*, 1696–1698.

Fisher, J. C. (1995, May 18). Stop scaring women. *USA Today*, p. 6.

Gabriel, S. E., O'Fallon, W. M., Kurland, L. T., Beard, C. M., Woods, J. E., & Melton, L. J. (1994). Risk of connective-tissue diseases and other disorders after breast implantation. *New England Journal of Medicine, 330*, 1697–1702.

Goodman, E. (1992, January 25). Weighing the still-unknown risks of implants. *St. Petersburg Times*, p. 16A.

Guthrie, R. H. (1994). *The truth about breast implants*. New York: John Wiley.

Hennekens, C. H., Lee, I., Cook, N. R., Hebert, P. R., Karlson, E. W., LaMotte, F., Manson, J., Buring, J. E. (1996). Self-reported breast implants and connective tissue diseases in female health professionals: A retrospective cohort study. *Journal of the American Medical Association, 275*, 616–621.

Iverson, R. E. (1991). National survey shows overwhelming satisfaction with breast implants. *Plastic and Reconstructive Surgery, 88*, 546–547.

Kessler, D. A., Merkatz, R. B., & Schapiro, R. (1993). A call for higher standards for breast implants. *Journal of the American Medical Association, 270*, 2607–2608.

Kolata, G. (1995, June 13). A case of justice, or a total travesty? *New York Times*, pp. D1, D5.

Kristof, K. (1995, May 23). Ripple effect: Dow Corning's decision to file for bankrupcy touches thousands of investors, bondholders and litigants. *Chicago Tribune,* p. C7.

Lack, A. (Executive Producer). (1990, December 10). *Face to face with Connie Chung.* New York: CBS.

Lu, L. B., Shoaib, B. O., & Patten, B. M. (1994). A typical chest pain syndrome in patients with breast implants. *Southern Medical Journal, 87,* 978–984.

Sanchez-Guerrero, J., Colditz, G. A., Karlson, E. W., Hunter, D. J., Speizer, F. E., & Liang, M. H. (1995). Silicone breast implants and the risk of connective-tissue diseases and symptoms. *New England Journal of Medicine, 332,* 1666–1670.

Spiers, E. M., Grotting, J. C., & Omura, E. F. (1994). An epidermal proliferative reaction associated with a silicone gel breast implant. *American Journal of Dermatopathology, 16,* 315–319.

Support for breast implants. (1994, December 1). *South China Morning Post,* p. 20.

Vasey, F. B., & Feldstein, J. (1993). *The silicone breast implant controversy: What women need to know.* Freedom, CA: Crossing Press.

Wells, A. F., Daniels, S., Gunasekaran, S., & Wells, K. E. (1994). Local increase in hyaluronic acid and interleukin-2 in the capsules surrounding silicone breast implants. *Annals of Plastic Surgery, 33,* 1–5.

Wells, K. E., Cruse, C. W., Baker, J. L., Daniels, S. H., Stern, R. A., Newman, C., Seleznick, H. J., Vasey, F. B., Brozena, S., Albers, S. E., & Fenske, N. (1994). The health status of women following cosmetic surgery. *Plastic and Reconstructive Surgery, 93,* 907–912.

Yoshidu, S. H., Teuber, S. S., German, J. B., & Gershwin, M. E. (1994). Immunotoxicity of silicone: Implications of oxidant balance towards adjuvand activity. *Food and Chemical Toxicology, 32,* 1089–1100.

CHAPTER 2

Brody, H. (1987). *Stories of sickness.* New Haven, CT: Yale University Press.

Brown, K. (1993, Fall). Logic of the psyche: Health care ethics and women's narrative. *From the Center: A Publication of the Center for Literature, Medicine, and the Health Care Professions, 3.*

Cousins, N. (1979). *Anatomy of an illness as perceived by the patient.* New York: W. W. Norton.

Crawford, R. (1984). A cultural account of "health": Control, release, and the social body. In J. B. McKinlay (Ed.), *Issues in the political economy of health care* (pp. 60–103). New York: Tavistock.

Fasching, D. (1989). *Religious ethics as narrative ethics.* Unpublished manuscript, University of South Florida, Tampa, Department of Religious Studies.

Fisher, W. R. (1984). Narration as a human communication paradigm: The case of public moral argument. *Communication Monographs, 51,* 1–22.

Fisher, W. R. (1985). The narrative paradigm: An elaboration. *Communication Monographs, 52,* 347–367.

Foss, S. K. (1989). *Rhetorical criticism: Exploration and practice.* Prospect Heights, IL: Waveland Press.

Gergen, K. J., & Gergen, M. M. (1983). Narratives of the self. In T. R. Sarbin & K. E. Scheibe (Eds.), *Studies in social identity* (pp. 254–273). New York: Praeger.

Holmes, H. B. (1989). Can clinical research be both ethical and scientific? *Hypatia, 4,* 154–165.

Jonsen, A. R., & Toulmin, S. (1988). *The abuse of casuistry.* Berkeley: University of California Press.

McAdams, D. P. (1993). *The stories we live by: Personal myths and the making of the self.* New York: Morrow.

Smith, D. H. (1993). Stories, values, and patient care decisions. In C. Conrad (Ed.), *The ethical nexus: Values in organizational decision making* (pp. 123–148). Norwood, NJ: Ablex.

Smith, D. H., & Occhipinti, S. L. (May, 1984). *Patient reactions to physician interviews.* Paper presented at the International Communication Association Convention, San Francisco.

Smith, D. H., & Pettegrew, L. S. (1986). Mutual persuasion as a model for doctor–patient communication. *Theoretical Medicine, 7,* 127–146.

Todd, A. D. (1989). *Intimate adversaries: Cultural conflict between doctors and women patients.* Philadelphia: University of Pennsylvania Press.

Vanderford, M. L., Smith, D. H., & Harris, W. S. (1992). Value identification in narrative discourse: Evaluation of an HIV education demonstration project. *Journal of Applied Communication Research, 20,* 123–160.

Young, I. M. (1990). *Throwing like a girl and other essays in feminist philosophy and social theory.* Bloomington: Indiana University Press.

Young, K. (1989). Narrative embodiments: Enclaves of the self in the realm of medicine. In J. Shotter & K. Gergen (Eds.), *Texts of identity* (pp. 152–165). Newbury Park, CA: Sage.

CHAPTER 3

Albrecht, T. L., & Adelman, M. B. (1984). Social support and life stress: New directions for communication research. *Human Communication Research, 11,* 3–32.

Arntson, P. (1989). Improving citizens' health competencies. *Health Communication, 1,* 29–34.

Arntson, P., & Droge, D. (1987). Social support in self-help groups: The role of communication in enabling perceptions of control. In T. L. Albrecht & M. B. Adelman (Eds.), *Communicating social support* (pp. 148–171). Newbury Park, CA: Sage.

Brody, H. (1987). *Stories of sickness.* New Haven, CT: Yale University Press.

Lack, A. (Executive Producer). (1990, December 10). *Face to face with Connie Chung.* New York: CBS.

Smith, D. H., & Pettegrew, L. S. (1986). Mutual persuasion as a model for doctor–patient communication. *Theoretical Medicine, 7,* 127–146.

Taylor, S. E. (1983). Adjustment to threatening events: A theory of cognitive adaptation. *American Psychologist, 38,* 1161–1173.

CHAPTER 4

Brody, H. (1987). *Stories of sickness.* New Haven, CT: Yale University Press.

Crawford, R. (1984). A cultural account of "health": Control, release, and the social body. In J. B. McKinlay (Ed.), *Issues in the political economy of health care* (pp. 60–103). New York: Tavistock.

Natanson, M. A. (1970). *The journeying self: A study in philosophy and social role.* Reading, MA: Addison-Wesley.

Young, I. M. (1990). *Throwing like a girl and other essays in feminist philosophy and social theory.* Bloomington: Indiana University Press.

CHAPTER 5

Berkel, H., Birdsell, D. C., & Jenkins, H. (1992). Breast augmentation: A risk factor for breast cancer? *New England Journal of Medicine, 326,* 1649–1653.

Ecklund, G. (1991, November). *Statement of the American College of Radiology and FDA Advisory Panel for general and plastic surgery devices.* Gaithersburg, MD: Food and Drug Administration.

Fisher, J. C. (1992). The silicone controversy—When will science prevail? *New England Journal of Medicine, 326,* 1696–1698.

Iverson, R. E. (1991). National survey shows overwhelming satisfaction with breast implants. *Plastic and Reconstructive Surgery, 88,* 546–547.

Sergent, J. S. (1992, February 27). Silicone gel breast implants and rheumatic disease. *Hotline: Newsletter of the American College of Rheumatology.*

CHAPTER 6

Altheide, D. L. (1974). *Creating reality.* Beverly Hills, CA: Sage.

Belson, A. A. (1983, August). Breast reconstruction: The second biggest decision for a mastectomy patient. *Ms.,* 96–98.

Breast implant maker fails to prove safety. (1991, November 14). *Tampa Tribune,* p. 11.

Capettini, R., & Towle, P. (1992, March 3). Dolly's breasts are killing her. *National Enquirer,* pp. 1, 31.

Carey, J. W. (1986). The dark continent of American journalism. In R. K. Manoff & M. Schudson (Eds.), *Reading the news* (pp. 146–196). New York: Pantheon.

Cowley, G., Springen, K., & Hager, M. (1992, January 20). Calling a halt to the big business of silicone implants. *Newsweek,* 56.

Craddock, J. (1992, March 7). Silicone scare taking a toll on surgeons. *St. Petersburg Times,* pp. 1B–2B.

Cruse, C. W., Novick, M., Brown, K., & Singer, K. (1991, April 23). More on breast implants (Letter to the Editor). *St. Petersburg Times,* p. 11A.

Davis, L. (1992, May). The implant panic. *Vogue,* pp. 166, 168, 170.

Eagan, A. B. (1992, July). The breast implant fiasco. *New Woman,* 123–127.

Epstein, E. J. (1973). *News from nowhere.* New York: Random House.

Firm to pay for implant removal. (1992, March 20). *St. Petersburg Times,* pp. 1A–2A.

Fischer, A. (1991, September). A body to die for. *Redbook,* 96–99, 173–174.

Fisher, W. R. (1984). Narration as a human communication paradigm: The case of public moral argument. *Communications Monographs, 51,* 1–22.

Freimuth, V. S., & Van Nevel, J. P. (1981). Reaching the public: The asbestos awareness campaign. *Journal of Communication, 31,* 155–167.

Gerbner, G., & Gross, L. P. (1976). Living with television: The violence profile. *Journal of Communication, 26,* 172–199.

Gross, J. (1991, November 5). Women with breast implant split on need for U.S. controls. *New York Times,* pp. A1, A11.

Gould, S., & Zucker, J. (Executive Producers). (1990, December 18). *NBC nightly news.* New York: NBC.

Gould, S., & Zucker, J. (Executive Producers). (1991a, April 14). *NBC nightly news.* New York: NBC.

Gould, S., & Zucker, J. (Executive Producers). (1991b, November 12). *NBC nightly news*. New York: NBC.

Haupt, D. E. (1987, May). Mastectomy treated Peggy McCann's cancer, but breast reconstruction made her well. *Life*, 78–83, 85–86, 88.

Implants likely to be much tougher to get. (1991, October 30). *St. Petersburg Times*, p. 3A.

James, S. (1991, February 17). Breast implants: How safe are they? *St. Petersburg Times*, pp. 1F, 10F.

James, S. (1992, March 18). Help for those with implants. *St. Petersburg Times*, 1D–2D.

Johnson, J. D., & Meischke, H. (1993). Cancer-related channel selection: An extension for a sample of women who have had a mammogram. *Women and Health, 20*, 31–44.

Jones, J. (1992, March 2). Body of evidence. *People*, 56–62.

Kee, F., Teleford, A. M., Donaghy, P., & O'Doherty, A. (1993). Enhancing mammography uptake: Who do women listen to? *European Journal for Cancer Prevention, 2*, 37–42.

Kilpatrick, J. J. (1992, January 25). Government's business is not breast implants (Editorial). *St. Petersburg Times*, p. 16A.

Landers, A. (1992, March 15). Breast implants are no cause for panic. *St. Petersburg Times*, p. 7F.

Manoff, R. K. (1986). Writing the news (by telling the story). In R. K. Manoff & M. Schudson (Eds.), *Reading the news* (pp. 197–229). New York: Pantheon.

Mason, D. (1992, January 18). Silicone breast implants: Now what? *St. Petersburg Times*, pp. 1D, 3D.

Mithers, C. L. (1992, April). Why women want man-made breasts. *McCall's*, 83–84, 86, 88, 90, 91, 141.

Nashner, M., & White, M. (1977, September). Beauty and the breast: A 60% complication rate for an operation you don't need. *Ms.*, 53–54, 84–85.

Panel advises restricting cosmetic breast implants. (1992, February 21). *St. Petersburg Times*, 1A–2A.

Peters, L. (1992, June). Beauty and the breast. *Redbook*, 84–87.

Quindlen, A. (1992, January 21). Breast implants: The real issue is safety (Editorial). *St. Petersburg Times*, p. 8A.

Regush, N. (1992, January/February). Toxic breasts. *Mother Jones*, 25–31.

Rigdon, J. E. (1992, March 20). Women find it difficult to get breast implants removed. *Wall Street Journal*, pp. B1, B10.

Ripley, J. (1992, February 24). Their double bond: Silicone and pain. *St. Petersburg Times*, p. 6B.

Rovner, S. (1991, January 22). Just how safe are silicone implants? *Washington Post*, p. 6.

Rybacki, K. C., & Rybacki, D. J. (1991). *Communication criticism: Approaches and genres*. Belmont, CA: Wadsworth.

Safety vs. self-esteem (Editorial). (1991, November 16). *St. Petersburg Times*, p. 20A.

Sanders, V. (1992, April). My twenty-year nightmare. *Ladies' Home Journal*, 20, 22, 24.

Scheer, R. (1991a, December 22). An escalating frenzy of lifts, nips, and tucks. *Los Angeles Times*, pp. A1, A42–A43.

Scheer, R. (1991c, December 24). Breast implant clients face maze of conflicting claims. *Los Angeles Times*, pp. A1, A10.

Seligmann, J. (1980, February 11). Building a new breast. *Newsweek*, 80.

Seligmann, J., & Church, V. (1992, March 2). A vote of no confidence. *Newsweek*, 75.

Seligmann, J., Cowley, G., & Springen, K. (1992, January 6). Another blow to implants. *Newsweek*, 45.

Singer, E., & Endreny, P. M. (1993). *Reporting on risk: How the mass media portray accidents, diseases, disasters, and other hazards*. New York: Russell Sage Foundation.

Sorensen, E. (Executive Producer). (1991, May 16). *CBS evening news*. New York: CBS.

Sorensen, E. (Executive Producer). (1992a, January 6). *CBS evening news*. New York: CBS.

Sorensen, E. (Executive Producer). (1992b, February 10). *CBS evening news*. New York: CBS.

Tuchman, G. (1978). *Making news*. New York: Free Press.

Vick, K. (1991, November 13). Women present favorable views on breast implants. *St. Petersburg Times*, p. 3A.

Weiner, S. L. (1986). Tampons and toxic shock syndrome: Consumer protection or public confusion? In H. M. Sapolsky (Ed.), *Consuming fears* (pp. 141–158). New York: Basic Books.

What price beauty? Plastic surgery under fire. (1992, June 8). *First for women*, 14–23.

CHAPTER 7

American Board of Family Practice. (1987). *Rights and responsibilities: Part II: The changing health care consumer and patient/doctor partnership*. Lexington, KY: Author.

Aristotle. (1932). *The rhetoric of Aristotle* (L. Cooper, Trans.). New York: Appleton-Century-Crofts.

Booming busts. (1991, January 12). *The Economist*, 81.

Byrne, J. A. (1992, February 24). Here's what to do next, Dow Corning. *Business Week*, 33.

Cowley, G., Springen, K., & Hager, M. (1992, January 20). Calling a halt to the big business of silicone implants. *Newsweek*, 56.

Craddock, J. (1992, March 7). Silicone scare taking a toll on surgeons. *St. Petersburg Times*, pp. 1B–2B.

Eagan, A. B. (1992, July). The breast implant fiasco. *New Woman*, 123–127.

Fischer, A. (1991, September). A body to die for. *Redbook*, 96–99, 173–174.

Fisher, W. R. (1984). Narration as a human communication paradigm: The case of public moral argument. *Communication Monographs, 51*, 1–22.

Golden, J. L., Berquist, G. F., & Coleman, W. E. (1989). *The rhetoric of western thought* (4th ed.). Dubuque, IA: Kendall/Hunt.

Harris & Associates. (1982). Views of informed consent and decision making: Parallel surveys of physicians and the public. In the President's Commission for the Study of Ethical Problems in Medicine and Biomedical and Behavioral Research, *Making health care decisions: The ethical and legal implications of informed consent in the patient–practitioner relationship* (pp. 17–316). Washington, DC: U.S. Government Printing Office.

James, S. (1991, February 17). Breast implants: How safe are they? *St. Petersburg Times*, pp. 1F, 10F.

James, S. (1992, March 18). Help for those with implants. *St. Petersburg Times*, pp. 1D–2D.

Jones, J. (1992, March 2). Body of evidence. *People*, 56–62.

Korsch, B. M., Gozzi, E. K., & Francis, V. (1968). Gaps in doctor–patient communication. *Pediatrics, 42*, 855–870.

Korsch, B. M., & Negrete, V. M. (1972). Doctor–patient communication. *Scientific American, 227*, 66–74.

McMahon, N. M. (1992, February 9). Can implants last forever? (Editorial). *Tampa Tribune*, p. 2.

Mechanic, D. (1968). *Medical sociology* (2nd ed.). New York: The Free Press.

Memos show problems with breast implants. (1992, February 11). *St. Petersburg Times*, pp. 1A–2A.

Mithers, C. L. (1992, April). Why women want man-made breasts. *McCall's*, 83–84, 86, 88, 90, 91, 141.

More action is needed in silicone-implant saga. (1992, March 20). *USA Today*, p. 8A.

Nashner, M., & White, M. (1977, September). Beauty and the breast: A 60% complication for an operation you don't need. *Ms.*, 53–54, 84–85.

Panel advises restricting cosmetic breast implants. (1992, February 21). *St. Petersburg Times*, 1A–2A.

Purvis, A. (1991, April 29). Time bombs in the breasts? *Time*, 70.

Regush, N. (1992, January/February). Toxic breasts. *Mother Jones*, 25–31.

Ripley, J. (1992, February 24). Their double bond: Silicone and pain. *St. Petersburg Times*, p. 6B.

Rovner, S. (1991, January 22). Just how safe are silicone implants? *Washington Post*, p. 6.

Sanders, V. (1992, April). My twenty-year nightmare. *Ladies' Home Journal*, 20, 22, 24.

Scheer, R. (1991b, December 23). Lack of regulations sparks cosmetic surgery turf war. *Los Angeles Times*, pp. A1, A28–A29.

Seligmann, J., & Church, V. (1992, March 2). A vote of no confidence. *Newsweek*, 75.

Seligmann, J., Hager, M., & Springen, K. (1992, March 23). Another tempest in a C cup. *Newsweek*, 67.

Seligmann, J., Yoffe, E., & Hager, M. (1991, April 29). The hazards of silicone. *Newsweek*, 56.

Todd, A. D. (1989). *Intimate adversaries: Cultural conflict between doctors and women patients.* Philadelphia: University of Pennsylvania Press.

Vick, K. (1991, November 13). Women present favorable views on breast implants. *St. Petersburg Times*, p. 3A.

Weiss, R. (1991, May 25). Implants: How big a risk? *Science*, 1060.

What price beauty? Plastic surgery under fire. (1992, June 8). *First for women*, 14–23.

CHAPTER 8

After U. S. warning, Dow curbs assurances about breast implants. (1992, January 1). *New York Times*, p. 8A.

Analysts: Dow must regain trust. (1992, February 12). *St. Petersburg Times*, p. 6A.

Breast implants: Assigning blame. (1992, January 27). *U. S. News and World Report*, 17.

Byrne, J. A. (1992, February 24). Here's what to do next, Dow Corning. *Business Week*, 33.

Cartoon. (1992, January 27). Perspectives. *Newsweek*, 15.

Castleman, M. (1991, March). The enemy within. *California Lawyer*, 44–48, 104–106.

Cowley, G., Springen, K., & Hager, M. (1992, January 20). Calling a halt to the big business of silicone implants. *Newsweek*, 56.

Dionisopoulos, G., & Vibbert, S. (1983, November). *Refining generic parameters: The case for organizational apologia.* Paper presented at the Speech Communication Association Convention, Washington, DC.

Dionisopoulos, G., & Vibbert, S. (1988). CBS vs. Mobil Oil: Charges of creative bookkeeping in 1979. In H.R. Ryan (Ed.), *Oratorical encounters* (pp. 241–251). Westport, CT: Greenwood.

Dow Corning. (1991, December 13). *Dow Corning and its employees call San Francisco jury award regarding breast implants "outrageous;" Characterize breast implant debate as sensationalistic and politicized* [Press release].

Dow Corning. (1992a, January 2). *Dow Corning calls Sid Wolfe claims "11th hour shadow boxing"* [Press release].

Dow Corning. (1992b, January 6). *Dow Corning Wright disagrees with FDA announcement; Urges agency to move regulatory process away from politics, back to science* [Press release].

Dow Corning. (1992c, January 10). *Remarks by Robert T. Rylee, Chairman, Health Care Businesses, Dow Corning Wright, National Press Club, Washington* [Company document].

Dow Corning. (1992d, January 13). *Dow Corning reaffirms safety of silicone breast implants; Amasses largest safety data base of any implantable medical device* [Press release].

Dow Corning. (1992e, February 10). Position statement on: Dow Corning Mammory Task Force. *Summary of scientific studies and internal company documents concerning silicone breast implants* [Company document].

Dow Corning. (1992f, March 19). *Dow Corning announces $10 million research fund to continue study of silicone breast implant safety; Affirms financial support for implant removal under certain conditions; And announces its withdrawal from the silicone breast implant market* [Press release].

Dow Corning. (1992g, March 6). *A chronology of key events: The silicone gel breast implant issue 1990–1992* [Company document].

Dow to stop making breast implants. (1992, March 19). *St. Petersburg Times*, p. 5A.

FDA: Hold off on silicone breast implant. (1992, January 7). *St. Petersburg Times*, pp. 1A, 8A.

Firm to pay for implant removal. (1992, March 20). *St. Petersburg Times*, pp. 1A–2A.

Friedman, P. (Executive Producer). (1991, December 31). *World news tonight with Peter Jennings*. New York: ABC.

Friedman, P. (Executive Producer). (1992, January 13). *World news tonight with Peter Jennings*. New York: ABC.

Galen, M., Byrne, J. A., Smart, T., & Woodruff, D. (1992, March 2). Debacle at Dow Corning: How bad will it get? *Business Week*, 36–38.

Goodman, E. (1992, January 25). Weighing the still-unknown risks of implants. *St.Petersburg Times*, p. 16A.

Gould, S., & Zucker, J. (Executive Producers). (1991, August 4). *NBC nightly news*. New York: NBC.

Gould, S., & Zucker, J. (Executive Producers). (1992a, January 13). *NBC nightly news*. New York: NBC.

Gould, S., & Zucker, J. (Executive Producers). (1992b, February 20). *NBC nightly news*. New York: NBC.

Gould, S., & Zucker, J. (Executive Producers). (1992c, March 18). *NBC nightly news*. New York: NBC.

Hearit, K. M. (1993, April). *Mistakes were made: The use of apologia in public relations crises*. Paper presented at Southern/Central States Communication Association Convention, Lexington, KY.

Hilts, P. J. (1992a, January 13). Maker of implants balked at testing, its records show. *New York Times*, pp. A1, B10.

Hilts, P. J. (1992b, February 19). Studies see greater implant danger. *New York Times*, p. A12.

Lack, A. (Executive Producer). (1990, December 10). *Face to face with Connie Chung*. New York: CBS.

Lawmaker seeks Dow Corning probe. (1992, February 17). *St. Petersburg Times*, p. 7A.

Mason, D. (1992, January 18). Silicone breast implants: Now what? *St. Petersburg Times*, pp. 1D, 3D.

McCue, P. S. (1993). Repealing Gibson's law. In J. Gottschalk (Ed.), *Crisis response: Inside stories on managing image under siege* (pp. 229–249). Detroit, MI: Gale Research.

McMillian, J. (1987). In search of the organizational persona: A rationale for studying organizations rhetorically. In L. Thayer (Ed.), *Organization-communication: Emerging perspectives II* (pp. 21–45). Norwood, NJ: Ablex.

Memos show problems with breast implants. (1992, February 11). *St. Petersburg Times*, pp. 1A–2A.

Quindlen, A. (1992, January 21). Breast implants: The real issue is safety. *St. Petersburg Times*, p. 8A.

Regush, N. (1992, January/February). Toxic breasts. *Mother Jones*, 25–31.

Reibstein, L., Washington, F., Tsaintor, D., & Hager, M. (1992, February 24). Fighting the implant fire. *Newsweek, 38.*

Seligmann, J., Cowley, G., & Springen, K. (1992, January 6). Another blow to implants. *Newsweek*, 45.

'74 study: Silicones affect immune system. (1992, January 18). *St. Petersburg Times*, p. 6A.

Smart, T. (1991, June 10). Breast implants: What did the industry know, and when Business Week, 94.

Sorenson, E. (Executive Producer). (1992a, January 13). *CBS evening news.* New York: CBS.

Sorenson, E. (Executive Producer). (1992b, February 18). *CBS evening news.* New York: CBS.

Walker, B. S. (1992, March 20). Implant pioneer bows out. *USA Today*, p. 1A.

Ware, B. L., & Linkugel, W. A. (1973). They spoke in defense of themselves: On the general criticism of apologia. *Quarterly Journal of Speech, 59,* 273–283.

CHAPTER 9

Berkel, H., Birdsell, D. C., & Jenkins, H. (1992). Breast augmentation: A risk factor for breast cancer? *New England Journal of Medicine, 326,* 1649–1653.

Council on Scientific Affairs. (1993). Silicone breast implants. *Journal of the American Medical Association, 270,* 2602–2606.

CHAPTER 10

Bantz, C. R. (1981). Public arguing in the regulation of health and safety. *Western Journal of Speech Communication, 45,* 71–87.

Berkel, H., Birdsell, D. C., & Jenkins, H. (1992). Breast augmentation: A risk factor for breast cancer? *New England Journal of Medicine, 326,* 1649–1653.

Bochner, A. P. (1994). Perspectives on inquiry II. In M. L. Knapp & G. R. Miller (Eds.), *Handbook of interpersonal communication* (pp. 21–41). Thousand Oaks, CA: Sage.

Boston Women's Health Book Collective. (1984). *The new our bodies, ourselves.* New York: Simon & Schuster.

Breast implant award upheld. (1995, January 10). *St. Petersburg Times*, p. 7A.

Brown, K. (1993, Fall). Logic of the psyche: Health care ethics and women's narrative. *From the Center: A publication of the Center for Literature, Medicine, and the Health Care Professions, 3.*

Conguergood, D. (1993). Storied worlds and the work of teaching. *Communication Education, 42,* 337–348.

Cowley, G., Hager, M., & Liu, M. (1994, May 16). Tracking the second storm. *Newsweek*, 56257.

Crawford, R. (1984). A cultural account of "health": Control, release, and the social body. In J. B. McKinlay (Ed.), *Issues in the political economy of health care* (pp. 60–103). New York: Tavistock.

Doctors resign from implant study. (1994, December 21). *St. Petersburg Times*, p. 4A.

Eraker, S. A., Kirscht, J. P., & Becker, M. H. (1984). Understanding and improving patient compliance. *Annals of Internal Medicine, 100,* 258–268.

For her, a state of civilized society is truly unbearable. (1994, November 8). *St. Petersburg Times*, p. 4A.

Friedman, P. (Executive Producer). (1991a, April 16). *World news tonight with Peter Jennings*. New York: ABC.

Friedman, P. (Executive Producer). (1991b, September 25). *World news tonight with Peter Jennings*. New York: ABC.

Friedman, P. (Executive Producer). (1992, February 9). *World news tonight with Peter Jennings*. New York: ABC.

Gosier, E. (1995, January 14). A basketball player dies of a heart defect, or could it have been a deadly disorder that afflicts tall people? *St. Petersburg Times*, p. 1B.

Gould, S., & Zucker, J. (Executive Producers). (1991, August 4). *NBC nightly news*. New York: NBC.

Gould, S., & Zucker, J. (Executive Producers). (1992a, January 5). *NBC nightly news*. New York: NBC.

Gould, S., & Zucker, J. (Executive Producers). (1992b, January 6). *NBC nightly news*. New York: NBC.

Gross, J. (1991, November 5). Women with breast implant split on need for U.S. controls. *New York Times*, pp. A1, A11.

Hilts, P. (1992c, February 19). Studies see greater implant danger. *New York Times*, p. A12.

Hitti, M. (1994, November 30). Tips on how to select a physician. *Atlanta Constitution*, p. E3. How is your doctor treating you? (1995, February). *Consumer Reports*, 81–88.

Korsch, B. M., Gozzi, E. K., & Francis, V. (1968). Gaps in doctor–patient communication. *Pediatrics*, *42*, 855–870.

Korsch, B. M., & Negrete, V. F. (1972). Doctor–patient communication. *Scientific American*, *227*, 66–74.

Mechanic, D. (1968). *Medical sociology* (2nd ed.). New York: The Free Press.

Molitor, F. (1993). Accuracy in science news reporting by newspapers: The case of aspirin for the prevention of heart attacks. *Health Communication*, *5*, 209–224.

Morris, L. A. (1990). *Communicating therapeutic risks*. New York: Springer-Verlag.

Ogur, B. (1984). *Long day's journey into night: Women and prescription drug abuse*. Unpublished manuscript. University of South Florida, Tampa.

Overreaction to implant controversy feared. (1992, April 18). *St. Petersburg Times*, p. 3A.

Panel advises restricting cosmetic breast implants. (1992, February 21). *St. Petersburg Times*, pp. 1A–2A.

Research on Gulf War Syndrome called "wasteful." (1995, January 5). *St. Petersburg Times*, p. 8A.

Rovner, S. (1991, January 22). Just how safe are silicone implants? *Washington Post*, p. 6.

Seligmann, J., & Church, V. (1992, March 2). A vote of no confidence. *Newsweek*, 75.

Singer, E., & Endreny, P. M. (1993). *Reporting on risk: How the mass media portray accidents, diseases, disasters, and other hazards*. New York: Russell Sage Foundation.

Smith, D. H. (1993). *Communication in medical practice*. University of South Florida, Tampa. Unpublished manuscript.

Sorenson, E. (Executive Producer). (1991, July 1). *CBS evening news*. New York: CBS.

Tennen, H., & Affleck, G. (1990). Blaming others for threatening events. *Psychological Bulletin*, *108*, 209–232.

Todd, A. D. (1989). *Intimate adversaries: Cultural conflict between doctors and women patients*. Philadelphia: University of Pennsylvania Press.

Author Index

219

Subject Index

Printed and bound by CPI Group (UK) Ltd, Croydon, CR0 4YY

17/10/2024

01775684-0007